D0803679

THE
MIRACLE OF
LEMONS

Dr Penny Stanway practised for several years as a GP and as a child-health doctor before becoming increasingly fascinated by researching and writing about a healthy diet and other natural approaches to health and wellbeing. She is an accomplished cook who loves eating and very much enjoys being creative in the kitchen and sharing food with others. Penny has written more than 20 books on health, food, and the connections between the two. She lives with her husband in a houseboat on the Thames and often visits the south-west of Ireland. Her leisure pursuits include painting, swimming and being with her family and friends.

THE MIRACLE OF LEMONS

Practical Tips for Health, Home & Beauty

DR. PENNY STANWAY

WATKINS PUBLISHING

LONDON

This edition first published in the UK and USA 2011 by
Watkins Publishing, Sixth Floor, Castle House,
75–76 Wells Street, London W1T 3QH

Designed and typeset by Paul Saunders
Printed in the U.S.A.

ISBN: 978-1-907486-48-7

In memory of Joan Rench, my much-loved mother, whose lemon meringue pie and lemon delicious were balm to the soul.

Contents

Acknowledgements

Thank you to my sister, Jenny Hare, for her joy in food and cooking; to my husband, Andrew, for his unstinting enthusiasm in discussing lemons; and to my agent, Doreen Montgomery, for her endless encouragement and support.

Introduction

Lemons are amazingly and enduringly popular. Their peel and juice have a delightfully fresh citrus aroma and a surprisingly sharp tang, and their wide variety of contents can help us care for our health, beauty and home, and flavour many foods and drinks. Lemons also have a great many commercial uses, such as in the production of flavourings and preservatives for soft drinks, foaming agents for detergents and solvents for paint-strippers.

Their astonishingly vibrant yellow colour, plus their shiny, grained surface and attractive ovoid shape, have inspired many artists to portray their beauty in paintings, ceramics, mosaics, reliefs, sculptures and fabrics. Some artists also use lemons as symbols of status (since they used to be very expensive), friendship, longevity and love.

On the more negative side, some artists use the image of a cut lemon to insinuate that something is sour, faulty or otherwise amiss. And in popular parlance, calling someone or something 'a lemon' suggests that all isn't as it should be. Certainly, lemons are nearly always extremely sour, because they contain a lot of acid but scarcely any sugar. However, this very acidity helps account for their domestic and commercial value, while a little culinary know-how makes them eminently edible and ensures their position among our favourite fruits.

CHAPTER ONE

The Lemon Tree

The evergreen lemon tree can grow up to 6m/19½ft high. Its fragrant blossoms are white inside, tinged with deep pink outside, and produced all year round. Every other year there is a large total crop of fruit, followed the next year by a lighter one. One tree can produce as many as 500–600 fruits a year (or even, from certain trees, up to 3,000 fruits) in several crops. The peak months for harvesting lemons in the Northern Hemisphere are May, June and August.

The average lemon weighs 75–150g/3–6oz. The heaviest recorded lemon in the world was grown in Israel in 2003 and weighed 5.2kg/11½lb). The lemon is one of the 16 species that make up the *Citrus* genus. Botanical historians believe that there were originally three species of *Citrus* tree: *Citrus medica* (the citron), *Citrus maxima* (the pomelo) and *Citrus reticulata* (the mandarin – including the tangerine, satsuma and clementine). The lemon tree (*Citrus limon*), as well as the orange (*Citrus sinensis*), grapefruit (*Citrus paradisi*), Persian lime (*Citrus latifolia*) and key lime (*Citrus aurantifolia*) and other types of citrus tree, originated from the various genetic crosses (hybridizations) of these three original species, or their offspring.

Citrus growers have developed about 47 varieties of lemon tree over many centuries of cultivation. However, lemons come in two main types: those that are relatively more acidic and those that are relatively sweeter. The most widely grown acidic varieties are the Eureka (the sourest lemon, large in size and with thick peel) and the Lisbon (medium-sized, with thin peel and no pips). The more acidic types are mainly grown commercially, whilst sweeter ones are mainly a domestic crop. One of the sweeter types, the Meyer 'lemon', is actually a lemon-mandarin hybrid, so is sweeter, juicier, rounder and less acidic than other lemons and has an orange-yellow colour.

Lemon trees grow best in semi-arid and arid subtropical regions of the world, and in temperatures that do not fall below 4°C/39°F. Lemon-producing countries include the USA (particularly California and Arizona), Mexico, Argentina, Chile, Brazil, Uruguay, Spain, Italy, Cyprus, Turkey, Israel, Syria, Iran, India, China, Morocco, Egypt, South Africa and Australia. More than 13 million tonnes of lemons are produced worldwide each year. However, it's difficult to be precise about lemon production because little published information is available, and because the Portuguese and Spanish word *limon* is the same for both the lemon and the lime.

The history of the lemon tree

Citrus trees are believed to have originated in central Asia, in the east Himalayan region of India, and Iran. The citrus trees that first came to Europe in the 2nd century were citron trees, which, although very aromatic, contain scarcely any juice. The lemon tree probably resulted from a cross between the citron and the lime, but when and where this happened is unknown. Lemon trees were well established in Iraq by the end of the 9th century and common in China and the Middle East by the 12th century. The Spanish and Portuguese took lemon seeds from there to Europe in the 15th century, Christopher Columbus took them to Haiti in 1493, and various Spanish adventurers introduced them to the Americas. The Dutch introduced them into South Africa by the middle of the 17th century, and the English took them to Australia in the late 18th century.

The word 'lemon' comes from the Middle English '*limon*', which in turn came from the Old French '*limon*', the Italian '*limone*', the Arabic '*laymun*' or '*limun*', the Persian '*limu*' and perhaps, originally, the Sanskrit '*nimbuka*'.

Cultivation

Lemon trees require:

- Warmth and sunshine – outdoors in a warm climate, or indoors in a heated greenhouse or a conservatory in a cooler climate.

- Protection from wind, which can prevent bees pollinating the flowers.

- Excellent drainage, so they should ideally be planted in a clay-free soil on slightly sloping ground.

- Regular feeding with citrus fertilizer (applied at the rate of 120g/4½oz for each year of the tree's age) in January,

May and September in the Northern Hemisphere and July, November and March in the Southern. Feed should be spread evenly below the leaf canopy, though not immediately around the trunk.

- Mulching to reduce competition from weeds and to prevent drying out.

- Regular watering, especially in dry weather and during flowering – particularly after pollination.

- Pruning to strengthen shoots, prevent crowding in the centre of the tree, keep the tree to an easily manageable height, and remove diseased and dead wood. Trimming the lower foliage reduces damage from snails and from fungi splashed up from the soil.

Pesticide use by commercial growers must adhere to their country's regulations. Domestic growers should take advice from a suitable handbook or from a nursery or garden centre. The latter two can also advise on the type of lemon tree that is most suitable for where you live, as trees vary in the cold-tolerance and disease-resistance of their rootstock.

CHAPTER TWO

What's in Lemons?

The lovely bright fruit of the lemon tree offers a tart and flavourful source of fibre, plus vitamin C and other nutrients. It also provides a wealth of other health-promoting substances, some of which occur in such riches in only a few other foods.

A lemon's four 'Ps'

A lemon has three layers: the peel (which cooks call the zest and botanists call the exocarp, epicarp or flavedo), the pith (mesocarp or albedo) and the pulp (endocarp or flesh). It also has pips, which are in its pulp.

- **Peel** This is the tough, shiny, textured, vibrant yellow (or green) outer layer. Depending on the variety of lemon and the growing conditions, the peel's thickness varies from a thin 1–2mm/1/16–1/8in to a thick 20cm/3/4in. Cellulose fibre makes up 30 per cent of the peel. Its other constituents include waxes, organic acids, carotenoid pigments and lemon oil. Tiny oil glands open via pores on to the surface of the peel.

- **Pith** This is the soft, spongy white lining of the peel. It's mainly composed of fibre but also contains small amounts of antioxidants (such as phenolic compounds and limonin) and other substances.

- **Pulp** This forms the inside of the lemon and is separated by fibrous membranes into eight to ten segments, each containing tiny ovoid sacs (vesicles) filled with pale yellow juice. This juice forms 20–25 per cent of the weight of a ripe lemon and contains 90 per cent of its vitamin C, as well as small amounts of other antioxidants, plus various vitamins, minerals and organic acids, and lemon oil.

- **Pips** These are the bitter, whitish seeds in the pulp of most lemons. Their contents include salicylic-acid salts (as in aspirin), limonin and a little lemon oil.

Lemons contain many health-promoting and otherwise useful substances, including nutrients, fibre, phenolic compounds, plant pigments, limonene, organic acids and limonoids.

Nutrients

Lemons are one of the best food sources of vitamin C (an antioxidant also known as ascorbic acid). The antioxidant properties and the acidity of lemons help to explain why they are so beneficial. One small (100g/3½oz) lemon contains 60–100mg of vitamin C. The recommended adult dietary allowance of this vitamin varies between countries, being 90mg a day in the US and 75mg in the UK, for example. So consuming one lemon a day can provide most, if not all, of your daily requirement. It's best to consume lemon juice freshly squeezed, as 20 per cent of its vitamin C is lost after eight hours at room temperature or 24 hours in a refrigerator.

Lemons also contain small amounts of sugar, plant pigments, beta carotene (also called 'pro-vitamin A', as the body makes it into this vitamin), vitamins B and E and minerals – particularly potassium, but also magnesium, phosphorus, calcium, copper, iron, manganese, selenium and zinc. Two-thirds of a lemon's iron is in its peel and pith; two-thirds of its calcium is in its juice. The amounts of vitamins and minerals are small but useful. Lemons also contain minute amounts of proteins and fats, and a medium-sized lemon contains 15 calories of energy.

Fibre

A lemon's peel, pith, pips and pulp membranes are rich in valuable dietary fibre (once called 'roughage' but now officially 'non-starch polysaccharides'). Lemons contain two types of fibre: cellulose, which strengthens cell walls, and pectin, which binds cells together.

Cellulose absorbs water in the digestive tract. This makes stools more bulky and less sticky, which helps to prevent constipation and diarrhoea.

Pectin dissolves in water in the digestive tract to form a gel. Pectin is an antioxidant (see page 8). About 90 per cent of dissolved pectin is fermented by the millions of 'good' bacteria in the large bowel, releasing butyric acid and other short-chain fatty acids. These acids are valuable to our health because they:

- Aid the absorption of calcium and other minerals from the bowel.

- Reduce the absorption of cholesterol from the bowel.

- Suppress the production of cholesterol by the liver while also boosting the proportion of HDL cholesterol (the 'good' type) in the blood.

- Encourage apoptosis ('suicide') of bowel-cancer cells.

Many people don't eat enough fibre. In the US, for example, the average intake is only half the recommended amount. Most of us could usefully increase our intake by including suitably prepared lemon peel and pith in recipes for foods and drinks.

Antioxidants

Lemons contain a wide variety of antioxidants, including many of their phenolic compounds (such as flavonoids and coumarins), as well as vitamins C and E, selenium, zinc, carotenoid pigments, limonin (which is different from limonene – see pages 13 and 18–20) and other limonoids, and pectin.

Antioxidants help to protect cholesterol and other body fats from being oxidized by unstable particles known as 'free radicals'. Your body makes more free radicals when it is physically stressed, such as if you smoke too much, expose yourself to too much sun or take too much exercise. The presence of oxidized fats in the body encourages sunburn, prematurely aged skin, infection, pregnancy problems (such as pre-eclampsia and miscarriage), eyesight problems (such as cataracts and age-related macular degeneration), gallstones, high blood pressure, heart attacks, memory loss, strokes and certain cancers.

What's more, studies suggest that a lemon's antioxidants

enhance the liver's ability to break down toxins by up to 35 per cent.

Many people hope that antioxidant supplements will help protect their health, and women are the biggest fans. But these supplements may behave differently to the antioxidants found in lemons and other foods. For example, certain studies show that eating vitamin-C-rich fruits and vegetables can reduce the damage to DNA (our cells' genetic material) that can trigger cancer, whilst certain other studies show that using vitamin-C supplements, do not have the same effect. Indeed, in 2002, a report in *The Lancet* of a five-year study at Oxford University found that people who took a daily supplement of the antioxidants beta carotene and vitamins C and E were no less likely than those who took a placebo ('dummy') supplement to develop either cancer or, indeed, heart attacks, strokes, asthma, cataracts, dementia or osteoporosis.

The good news is that most of us can get all the antioxidants we need from a healthy diet that contains at least five helpings of vegetables and fruit a day – and lemons are an excellent source.

If you need more antioxidants than usual – for example, in later life, or if you have an infection, feel stressed, or smoke (one cigarette destroys 25mg of the body's vitamin C) – the solution is to eat more antioxidant-rich foods. Including lemons in your diet will give you a great start.

Phenolic compounds

These are present mainly in a lemon's peel and in smaller amounts in its pith and juice. Derived from phenolic acid, and also called polyphenols, their levels vary according to the variety of lemon tree, the maturity of the fruit, the geographical region (because of differing soil chemistry) and the year (because of changing climatic conditions). They include certain flavonoids and coumarins.

Many phenolic compounds are antioxidants and some are even more effective than vitamin C.

Flavonoids

These are water-soluble compounds that have also been called citrin, bioflavonoids and vitamin P. The flavonoids in lemons and other citrus fruits are the most biologically active of all the flavonoids in the edible plant kingdom. The highest concentration is in a lemon's peel and pith. Many lemon flavonoids are antioxidants and some are the yellow pigments that help to give lemon peel its sunny colour. Examples include diosmine, eriocitrin, hesperidin, limotricine, naringin, nobiletin, quercetin and tangeretin.

Some of a lemon's antioxidant flavonoids – the polymethoxylated flavones (PMFs) – are dubbed 'super-flavonoids'. The most common are nobiletin and tangeretin. A lemon's peel is 20 times richer than its juice in PMFs.

Studies suggest that flavonoids have many health benefits:

- They guard the power of vitamin C by improving its absorption and protecting it from oxidation.

- Super-flavonoids reduce LDL cholesterol (the potentially damaging type) by up to 40 per cent, possibly by reducing its production in the liver.

- A high intake is associated with a reduced risk of heart disease.

- They strengthen the walls of our capillaries (tiny blood vessels), so maximizing their potential volume and encouraging good blood flow.

- Their antioxidant power can discourage cancer. For example, naringenin helps to prevent DNA damage and enhances DNA repair.

Hesperidin is one of the most intensively studied antioxidant flavonoids. It can strengthen capillaries, reduce cholesterol and blood pressure, help maintain bone density, discourage overwhelming infection, have anti-inflammatory and sedative effects, and penetrate the blood–brain barrier (implying it can help to protect the brain from infection or other inflammation). Naringin is a particularly bitter-tasting antioxidant flavonoid, which scientists believe can also help to lower cholesterol.

Another flavonoid, rutin (known in its slightly different form as quercetin), is found in lemon peel and reported to bind ('chelate') potentially harmful heavy metals, so aiding their expulsion from the body.

Coumarins

These are phenolic compounds and their concentrations in a lemon's peel (and mainly in its oil) are up to 100 times higher than in its pulp. They include auraptene, bergamotene, isopimpinellin, limettin, certain psoralens (such as oxypeucedanin, and 5-methoxypsoralen – also known as bergapten), scopoletin and umbelliferone.

Some coumarins can benefit our health because they are

antioxidants. For example, studies suggest that auraptene helps prevent degenerative diseases and cancer.

Certain psoralens in lemons can be a problem because they are photoactive. This means that putting lemon oil on the skin makes it extra-sensitive to sunlight. Such photosensitivity can cause either phototoxicity or photo-allergy:

- Phototoxicity produces rapid sunburn that can last for weeks and permanently stain the skin.

- Photo-allergy produces dermatitis (skin inflammation) caused by an immunological reaction transforming a particular skin protein into an antigen ('allergen'). It occurs only in genetically predisposed people who are already sensitized. The rash usually resembles eczema, though there can be uricarial wheals (hives or 'nettle-rash') or hard, thick, itchy patches (lichenoid lesions). The rash can extend to skin that hasn't been in the sun. It resolves if sunlight is avoided.

You can protect yourself from a photosensitive reaction. For example, if you have a massage using a product containing lemon oil, avoid sunlight for 12 hours afterwards. Alternatively, ensure that only one drop of lemon oil in every two teaspoons of carrier oil are used for the massage. And if you zest a lemon, wear rubber gloves or wash your hands afterwards.

Pigments

A lemon's pigments are mainly in its peel. They include carotenoids (orange carotenes, such as beta carotene, and yellow xanthophylls, such as lutein, zeaxanthin, beta cryptoxanthin);

green chlorophylls; and yellow flavonoids. As a lemon ripens, its colour changes from green to yellow as a result of the hormone-controlled replacement of chlorophylls with carotenoids. Lemon pigments promote health. For example:

- High levels of carotenoids in the blood discourage heart disease by helping prevent the oxidation of fats. In particular, they help prevent the oxidation of LDL cholesterol (the potentially damaging sort), and thereby help keep arteries healthy and blood flowing freely.

- Beta carotene and beta cryptoxanthin are converted in the body into vitamin A, which promotes eye health and discourages infection.

Limonin

This and other limonoids (such as nomilin) are antioxidants that belong to a family of substances called terpenoids. Limonin is found throughout a lemon, though mainly in its pith and pips. It is present in about the same amount as vitamin C. Most people say it tastes very bitter. Studies show that limonoids can help prevent cell multiplication in cancers of the mouth, skin, lung, breast, stomach and colon. What's especially interesting is that limonin lasts in the body for up to 24 hours, whereas most other anti-cancer agents in foods remain for much less time. Scientists also suspect that limonin helps prevent the production of LDL cholesterol (the potentially dangerous sort) in the liver.

Organic acids

The acids in lemons include ascorbic acid (vitamin C) (see pages 6–7), citric acid (about 5 per cent of the juice) and glucaric acid. Lemons taste sour because they contain too little sugar to mask their acidity. Most of the acidity is in the juice – and its pH of 2.1 makes this even more acidic than vinegar at pH 2.4–3. (The pH indicates a liquid's acidity or alkalinity: 7 is neutral; below 7 is increasingly acid; above 7 is increasingly alkaline.)

Lemon acids can aid digestion in people who don't make enough of their own gastric acid. After the contents of a lemon or its juice have been digested, the lemon acids are metabolized (broken down) into water and carbon dioxide. The breakdown of the other contents releases alkalizing minerals (calcium, iron, magnesium, potassium, sodium). In contrast, most other fruits (including apples, bananas, grapes, oranges, pears, pineapples) contain so much sugar that their metabolism adds to the body's acid load.

Rubbing lemon juice over the cut surfaces of fruits and vegetables such as apples and potatoes stops them going brown. This is because the lemon acids inhibit an enzyme called polyphonoloxidase, which oxidizes phenolic compounds and turns them brown.

Lemon juice can prevent fish from smelling unpleasant because its acids neutralize protein breakdown products called amines in fish flesh. It can also tenderize fish and meat because its acids alter a tough protein called collagen in the flesh.

Historically, some women around the Mediterranean aimed to prevent pregnancy by soaking a piece of sea-sponge in a mixture of one part of lemon juice to five parts of water and putting it in their vagina before sex. This would have added to

the natural acidity of the vagina. The DNA in sperm is n
protected from being broken down by the vagina's acidity,
thanks to substances called amines in seminal fluid, which make
semen alkaline. But extra acidity from diluted lemon juice can
overwhelm this protection and stop sperm swimming in as
short a time as 30 seconds, so they can't get to the egg and
fertilize it. However, while this might sound like a useful method
of contraception, experts consider it unacceptably unreliable
compared with modern methods of contraception.

Citric acid

This is one of the alpha hydroxy acids (AHAs) beloved of
beauty-product manufacturers. Skin products containing
AHAs have moisturizing and exfoliating properties, as they
help the skin retain water and encourage the separation of
dead skin cells. This explains why applying lemon juice can
moisturize dry skin and restore softness and smoothness to
hard, cracked or flaking skin.

Consuming the citric acid in lemon juice helps move any
excess water from the body's tissues into the bloodstream. This
reduces congestion in the tissues and enables the blood to flow
more freely.

Citric acid is also used in foods and drinks as a preservative
and a flavouring (denoted in Europe by the 'E number' E330).
It is also put in soaps and laundry detergents (as it makes them
foam and work better in hard water), water-softeners, bathroom and kitchen cleaning products, effervescent medications,
cosmetics, bath salts and bath 'bombs', and shampoos that
remove wax and colouring from hair. It is also used to make
concrete set more slowly!

Glucaric acid

This could have important health benefits, as research suggests that it helps to:

- Lower LDL cholesterol (the potentially damaging sort) by up to 35 per cent, but doesn't affect HDL cholesterol (the protective sort).

- Discourage bowel cancer and inflammatory bowel disease by promoting butyric-acid production in the large bowel.

- Prevent oestrogen-sensitive cancer of the breast, prostate, ovary and colon, achieved by suppressing the enzyme beta-glucuronidase. This suppression enables a process called glucuronidation in the liver, which makes oestrogen more water-soluble and so aids its elimination in the urine.

- Prevent pre-menstrual syndrome by encouraging glucuro-nidation (above).

- Rid the body of pollutants by encouraging glucuronidation (above).

Lemon oil

This pale yellow or green oil, also known as 'lemon essential oil', forms 6 per cent of the weight of a lemon's peel; much smaller amounts are also present in the juice and pips. It takes around 3,000 lemons to produce 1kg/2lb 4oz of lemon oil. Enormous volumes of lemon oil are used commercially, for example in soft drinks (such as sodas, lemonades, squashes), foods, soaps, detergents, perfumes and medicines.

Lemon oil has around 300 constituents, including:

- Terpenes – mainly limonene (this forms 90 per cent of the oil; see below), but also citral (5 per cent of the oil; see page 20) and traces of citronellal, farnesenes, geraniol, linalool, myrcene, nerol, nootkatone, pinene, sabinene, terpinene and terpineol.

- Flavonoids, such as diosmin and limotricine.

- Coumarins, such as bergamotene and limettine.

- Hydrocarbons, such as benzanthracene, cymene and sinensal.

- Alcohols, such as nonanol and octanol.

- Aldehydes, such as decanal.

- Methyl anthranilate, which smells strongly of grapes.

- Waxes.

The composition of lemon oil varies according to the type of tree and soil. The extraction method that least alters the oil is cold-pressing, followed by spinning, but the oil may also be:

- Distilled to remove its terpenes; terpene-free oil keeps better and has more aroma as it has a higher concentration of aldehydes.

- Steam-distilled to remove its coumarins and to produce limonene. The resulting oil is psoralen-free, so it can't trigger photosensitive skin reactions.

- Adulterated with synthetic limonene, citral or dipentene.

- Concentrated.

- Treated with preservatives such as BHA (butylated hydroxyanisole) or BHT (butylated hydroxytoluene) to prolong its shelf life.

- Diluted with cheaper oil, such as orange or lime. Orange oil, for example, is ten times cheaper yet contains much the same ingredients, albeit in different percentages (for example, it has much less terpineol).

Lemon oil stimulates the gut and pancreas and, thanks mainly to its limonene content, has antibacterial, antiviral and antifungal properties. It is said to be soothing, relaxing, hypnotic, sedative and anti-inflammatory and also to stimulate the circulation.

When blended with other oils, lemon oil provides a 'top' fragrance note. Its scent is said to lift the spirits, clear the mind and improve concentration. Indeed, the number of typing mistakes halved in a Japanese study in which its vapour was diffused through an office.

Lemon oil should be kept in the dark and used within eight to ten months of opening, since light and air oxidize it, making it cloudy and unpleasant smelling. You can buy lemon oil from various pharmacies and other shops, and online.

Limonene

This (known in a slightly different form as dipentene) is the major component of lemon oil, and a little leaches into the juice. Limonene is a colourless liquid terpene that tastes bitter and smells strongly of oranges. However, its scent is masked by those of other odoriferous compounds in lemon oil – especially by the lilac scent of terpineol (a main fragrance ingredient in lapsang souchong tea, originating from the pine smoke that dried the tea).

Limonene produced by the steam-distillation of lemon oil is used as a flavouring and dietary supplement as well as in fragrances, cosmetic products, medicines and insecticides. It's also a good general-purpose solvent, hence its use in paint-strippers and cleaning products.

Our limonene intake depends on our diet. For example, the average daily limonene intake from food in the US as a whole is 16mg but in Arizona it is 70–130mg from citrus fruit alone.

Limonene has important health benefits. For example, it floats on the stomach contents, so if these reflux into the gullet, limonene coats the gullet lining, protecting it from damage by stomach acid. Limonene also speeds stomach emptying, which discourages acid reflux and other causes of indigestion; and it makes a barrier to bacteria that might infect the lining of the stomach and gut.

Limonene also has anti-cancer actions, according to studies that suggest it reduces the incidence and size of certain cancers. In particular, it can:

- Inhibit the cell divisions responsible for stomach, lung, liver and breast cancer; for example, limonene inhibits breast cancer in rats when given pure or as orange oil.

- Encourage a process in the liver called glucuronidation, which aids the elimination from the body of carcinogens (cancer-causing chemicals) and excess oestrogen (associated with oestrogen-dependent cancers of the breast, prostate and bowel).

- Encourage apoptosis ('suicide') of stomach-cancer cells.

- Boost immunity – for example, by encouraging white blood cells to kill cancer cells.

Certain researchers now consider limonene to be a significant anti-cancer agent with potential value as a dietary anti-cancer tool.

Citral

Also known as lemonal, this is the second biggest component of lemon oil. It comprises two terpenoid aldehydes, geranial and neral. These are isomers (meaning virtually identical to each other) and different from two of the other constituents of lemons called geraniol and nerol.

Citral has several possible health benefits. For one thing, it has antimicrobial qualities. For another, studies show that it encourages a process in the liver called glucuronidation – which helps rid the body of unwanted pollutants, hormones and carcinogens.

Lemon scent and flavour

A lemon's wonderful complex fragrance results from the combination of the fragrances of its many scented components. These are mainly terpenes (many of whose names end in 'ene') and their derivatives – including various alcohols (whose names end in 'ol') and aldehydes (whose names end in 'al'). There are also various coumarins and unsaturated fatty acids. The compounds that contribute most to a lemon's odour are citral, limonene, pinene and terpinene. One of the main reasons for the difference in scent of various lemon oils is their ratio of citral to citronellal.

A lemon's fragrance components include:

- bergamotene (black pepper)

- bisabolene (sweet, spicy, balsamic)

- cadinene (woody)

- camphene (pungent)

- caryophyllene (musky, oriental, sandalwood)

- citral (lemon)

- citronellal ('green', citrus)

- decanal (orange)

- dipentene (pine, lime, herbal, lemon)

- farnesenes (apple)

- geranial (strong lemon)

- geraniol (rose)

- heptanal (fresh, 'green', citrus)

- hexanol (herbaceous, woody)

- limonene (orange)

- linalool (sweet, woody, lavender)

- methyl anthranilate (grape)

- myrcene (woody)

- neral (sweet lemon)

- nerol (sweet rose)

- nonanol (fresh, spicy, herbaceous)

- nootkatone ('green', grapefruit)

- octanal (citrus)

- paracymene (fresh, citrus, woody, spicy)

- phellandrene (peppery, minty, citrus)

- pinene (pine, resinous)

- sabinene (marjoram)

- scopoletin (oaky, nutty)

- terpinene ('green', citrus)

- terpineol (lilac)

- umbelliferone (woody, medicinal)

The taste of a lemon comes from its acids, its various bitter principles – including limonene (found mainly in a lemon's oil) and limonin, the flavonoid naringin (found mostly in the pith and pips) and its tiny amounts of sugar. The presence of these sour, bitter and sweet substances in saliva is picked up by taste-receptor nerve endings in the taste buds of the tongue and various other parts of the mouth. A few people are genetically unable to detect bitterness in lemons and other foods.

Other plants with a lemon scent or flavour include lemon balm, lemon geranium, lemon grass, lemon myrtle, lemon verbena and lemon-scented varieties of basil, mint and thyme. My favourite flower scent – that of the large waxy blossoms of *Magnolia grandiflora* – is lemony too.

Added wax, pesticide and other substances

Most lemon farmers spray their trees with pesticides, such as fungicides and insecticides. They may also spray on a growth regulator to make the lemons larger, and spray the ground around the trees with a herbicide to get rid of weeds. Pesticide residues on lemons are washed off in the packing house along with dirt and the lemons' natural wax coating. However, pesticide residues may remain within the lemon's pulp.

Most harvested lemons are sprayed with a water-based emulsion containing wax, a fungicide and, perhaps, a bactericide, a preservative and other substances. The wax helps prevent the loss of moisture and aroma. It also reduces damage during handling, storage and transportation, makes lemons look glossy and accentuates their colour. It may be plant-, insect-, animal- or petroleum-based; carnauba palm wax is the most common.

Other compounds sometimes sprayed on after harvesting include ethyl alcohol (to improve the consistency of the wax), casein (to help the wax form an even film) and soap (to aid the flow of the spray).

Unripe green lemons are then stored in climate-controlled conditions for up to 20 weeks, and ripe yellow ones for six weeks.

Lemons are sometimes packed in paper wraps, pads or box liners impregnated with diphenyl fungicicide. This is taken up by a lemon's rind but not by its pulp.

The pesticides and herbicides permitted for use on lemons vary from country to country. The fungicides used might include benomyl, carbendazim, diphenyl, imazalil, orthophenyl phenol, thiabendazole, prochloraz, pyraclostrobin, pyridaben, pyrimethanil. Insecticides might include bromopropylate, chlorpyrifos, methidathion, pyriproxifen. An example of a herbicide is 2,4-dichlorophenoxyacetic acid; an example of a bactericide is orthophenyl phenol.

Many countries test samples of lemons to check that any traces of pesticides and other added chemicals, both on their surface and inside them, are within maximum permitted levels (MPL). If so, the fruit is deemed safe to eat.

In the UK, for example, in 2009, the Pesticide Residues Committee (an independent expert group that oversees the government's pesticide residues surveillance programme) arranged tests for up to 230 pesticide residues on and in 55 samples (11 from the European Union, and 44 from outside). Whilst 49 samples contained pesticide residues, and 47 contained more than one pesticide, none had residues in excess of the MPL.

In the US, pesticide residues are monitored by the Department of Agriculture Pesticide Data Program.

Washing a lemon (see pages 89–90) before consuming it reduces pesticide traces on the peel but not inside the lemon.

Alternatively, you may prefer to buy organic and unwaxed lemons. Depending on each country's regulations, there has generally either been no use of pesticides on lemons allowed to be labelled 'organic', or at least no routine use.

CHAPTER THREE

Natural Remedies

Lemons have long been prized as an aid to health. Their health-giving components include antiseptics, antifungals, antivirals, diuretics, astringents, tonics, antioxidants, detoxifiers, anti-cancer agents, anti-inflammatories and antihistamines. Traditional use, common sense and anecdotal evidence suggest that lemons can help many different ailments, but few scientific trials have been done because funding is problematic as lemons and their components cannot be patented.

The dictionary of ailments in this chapter details how and why lemons can help, but don't forget that you can also discourage common ailments with a healthy diet, adequate hydration, regular exercise, daily outdoor light, effective stress management, a sensible alcohol intake and no smoking.

The strategies outlined should not take the place of medical diagnosis and therapy. Avoid lemons if you are allergic to them. Also, note that their acidity may temporarily soften tooth enamel, making it vulnerable to damage, so dilute their juice and either use a straw to consume drinks containing lemon juice or rinse your mouth with water afterwards. Also, don't brush your teeth soon after you have finished the drink, as this might cause micro-abrasions of your softened tooth enamel.

When including lemon juice and zest in your diet, remember that you can take them in water, lemonade or a wide variety of foods, including salad dressings, sauces, salsas, soups, casseroles, grills, cakes, breads and pies. You can also cook lemon slices with fish and roast the empty 'shells' of squeezed lemons with vegetables or meat, as cooking softens the rind.

When a study is mentioned along with the name of the journal and the year of publication, this, plus some keywords, should enable you to find out more on the Internet.

Ailments and remedies

Acne

One possible cause is over-production of sebum caused by oversensitivity of sebaceous glands to testosterone. Others include changes in sebum, and unusually sticky hair-follicle cells. Triggers include the pre-menstrual fall in oestrogen, humidity, stress, certain drugs (for example, the progestogen-only Pill) and polycystic ovary syndrome. A reduction in the skin's acidity may encourage infection with acne bacteria.

Lemon juice may help because it kills acne bacteria, increases skin acidity, 'cuts' (emulsifies) skin oil and reduces inflammation.

Action: Apply lemon juice with a cotton pad 2 or 3 times a day.

Age spots

The most common are brown age freckles caused by normal ageing plus photo-ageing (accelerated ageing from sun-exposure).

Some people say lemon juice lightens age spots.

Action: Apply lemon juice each day, and the spots may begin to lighten within 6 weeks.

Include the zest and juice of a lemon in your daily diet, as their antioxidants may delay age freckles and other signs of ageing of the skin.

Ageing

Elderly people absorb less nourishment, which can contribute to premature ageing. Indeed, a recent UK survey noted that one in ten over-65s were short of iron and vitamins B and C, all of which lemons can help provide. Studies suggest that antioxidants discourage premature ageing of the skin. Vitamin C and other antioxidants in lemons might help counter premature ageing elsewhere in the body, too – for example, in joints and blood vessels. What's more, in Westernized cultures lemon acids could help the one in two over-60s who have an age-related reduction in stomach acid, because this makes many of them unable to absorb certain nutrients properly.

US researchers say that certain mineral and vitamin deficiencies accelerate age-related decay of mitochondria (the energy-providing structures in cells).

Molecular Aspects of Medicine, 2005

Scientists have long searched for lifestyle factors that encourage long life and discourage age-related diseases such as arthritis, heart disease, diabetes, cancer, osteoporosis and Alzheimer's. Long-lived peoples include certain groups in Russia, Pakistan, Ecuador, China, Tibet and Peru. One link is that many live at high altitudes, where glacier water is rich in alkaline minerals such as calcium. Such minerals help the body maintain a healthy pH (acid–alkaline balance) without drawing calcium from the bones. Lemon juice can have a similar effect.

Another factor linking many of these long-lived peoples is their consumption of lactic and acetic acids from fermented vegetables, fruit, milk, cereal grain, sugars, meat and fish. Like lemon acids, these help the body maintain a healthy pH.

Consuming vinegar before a meal discourages high blood sugar afterwards. Experts say the acids in lemon juice mean it's likely to behave in the same way.

The antioxidants in lemons may also reduce the inflammation associated with heart disease, arthritis and Alzheimer's. Lemon consumption may also discourage certain cancers, and strokes. It's said that the vitamin C a person gets by consuming lemon juice each day can raise their life expectancy by 6 years.

Finally, pectin encourages the elimination of toxic heavy metals, such as aluminium and lead, in the gut (and is prescribed for this purpose in Russia). Such metals encourage premature degeneration and ageing of brain and other cells. A lemon's peel, pith and segment walls are rich in pectin.

Action: Include the zest and juice of a lemon in your daily diet.

Alzheimer's disease

This condition destroys brain cells and is associated with patches of amyloid protein and clusters of tangled nerve fibres in the brain. Experts believe that inflammation is partly to blame. Also, research suggests that damage from oxidation of the brain's two most abundant polyunsaturated fatty acids – docosahexaenoic acid and arachidonic acid – contributes to Alzheimer's. Finally, affected people have high levels of the amino acid homocysteine. A lack of B vitamins raises homo-cysteine levels, and sufferers are particularly likely to go short of these vitamins. Lemons may help, as they contain antioxi-dants, other anti-inflammatories and B vitamins.

Laboratory tests in the US and Korea reveal that the antioxidant quercetin helps protect rat brain cells from oxidation.

Journal of Agricultural and Food Chemistry, 2004

Lemons contain anti-inflammatories such as hesperidin, which can penetrate the blood–brain barrier.

Journal of Neurochemistry, 2003

Action: Include the zest and juice of a lemon in your daily diet.

Anaemia

Iron-deficiency anaemia can be associated with low levels of stomach acid. This reduces iron absorption from food; it can also be associated with vitamin B_{12}-deficiency anaemia. Low stomach acid affects one in two over-60s and can result from ageing, stress, the prolonged use of acid-suppressant medication, and an unhealthy diet high in meat, grain, sugar and carbonated drinks (which produce acid in the body) but low in vegetables and fruits.

In someone who lacks stomach acid, a lemon's acidity could aid digestion by lowering the pH of the stomach.

Some alternative practitioners suggest, though without proof, that sodium from fruits and vegetables could help prevent the body diverting sodium from stomach-acid-producing cells and thus reducing stomach acid. They say this frees sodium to 'partner' acids in the urine and thereby remove excess acidity from the body.

In addition, a lemon's pectin is broken down by gut bacteria, releasing short-chain fatty acids, which boost iron absorption by raising acidity.

Action: Drink a glass of water containing 2 teaspoons of lemon juice before each meal.

Ankle swelling

The flavonoid rutin in lemons strengthens vein walls, so may reduce ankle swelling caused by fluid seeping from varicose veins. Lemons may also ease any fluid retention associated with heart or kidney disease because they have diuretic action – meaning they increase urine production.

Action: Include the zest and juice of a lemon in your daily diet.

Anxiety

Eating lemons might reduce anxiety or even panic attacks.

Researchers say that the urine of people with panic attacks is unusually acidic.

Psychiatry Research, 2005

Unusually acidic urine suggests that the kidneys are trying to prevent threatened over-acidity of the body. One reason could be an unbalanced diet with a lot of grain, sugar and meat but insufficient vegetables and fruit. Lemons can help the body maintain its normal pH (acid–alkaline balance).

Action: Consume the juice of one or two lemons each day.

Arthritis

Inflammation links most kinds of arthritis. Lemon antioxidants help reduce inflammation. Some people believe they should avoid lemons because they are acidic. But we metabolize lemon acids to potassium carbonate, which helps prevent excess acidity in our body.

Hesperidin, concentrated in lemon pith, is an anti-inflammatory antioxidant, so may reduce joint inflammation.
Journal of Pharmacy and Pharmacology, 1994

A study of more than 20,000 subjects who kept diet diaries and were arthritis-free when the study began, indicates that vitamin C-rich foods such as lemons can help protect against inflammatory polyarthritis, a form of rheumatoid arthritis involving two or more joints. This arthritis was more than three times as likely in those who consumed the least vitamin C-rich food as in those who ate the most.
Annals of Rheumatic Diseases, 2004

Action: Include the zest and juice of a lemon in your daily diet.

Massage joints with 1 drop each of lemon and pine oils in 2 teaspoons of sweet almond or other carrier oil.

Asthma

Inflammation and oversensitivity of the airways causes wheezing, a cough and tightness of the chest. Triggers include cold air, exercise, certain foods, hormone changes, laughter, infection, fumes, suddenly reduced air-pressure, thunderstorms, allergy and rapid breathing.

Lemons contain anti-inflammatory antioxidants. One of these, quercetin, also acts as an antihistamine.

In 1931, Dr George W. Bray of The Hospital for Sick Children, London, measured stomach acid after a meal in more than 200 children with asthma. Astonishingly, 9 per cent had none, 48 per cent had a severe lack and 23 per cent had a slight lack. So four in five lacked sufficient stomach acid! Other researchers have found a lack of stomach acid in many adults with asthma. One possible cause of allergic sensitization of the lining of the airways is absorption from the gut into the blood of poorly digested protein particles – which can be associated with low stomach acid. This is extraordinarily interesting but largely ignored. It's possible for low stomach acid to be encouraged by an acid-producing diet rich in grain, sugars, meat, dairy and carbonated drinks and low in fruit and vegetables. Some alternative practitioners suggest, though without proof, that a deficiency of sodium from fruits and vegetables encourages the body to remove sodium from various places – including stomach-acid-producing cells – so it's available to escort acid from the body in the urine. They say this could reduce stomach acid production.

Action: If you suspect that you have low stomach acid (for example, because you get indigestion unrelieved by antacids), try taking 2 teaspoons of lemon juice three times a day to help prevent asthma.

Alternatively, take lemon juice early in an attack. For an adult, put 1 tablespoon of lemon juice in a glass of water and sip it over half an hour. Wait for half an hour, then repeat. For a child, use less, depending on their size. Asthma medication prescribed by a doctor should also be taken.

Athlete's foot

This fungal infection between the toes is often picked up around swimming pools. Anecdotal reports suggest that lemon juice might help.

Action: Soak a cotton pad in lemon juice and apply to the affected area. Alternatively, bathe feet in a bowl of water containing 2 tablespoons of lemon juice.

Bites and stings

Wasp stings irritate because they are alkaline, so lemon acids may help. They may also ease irritation from mosquito and gnat bites.

Action: For a wasp sting or mosquito or gnat bites, apply a cotton pad soaked in lemon juice, and repeat if necessary.

Bronchitis

Chronic bronchitis is an obstructive lung disease that may require ever-more intensive treatment. Anti-inflammatory antioxidants seem to be protective, and quercetin may play a key role. Pectin may help too.

Researchers say that high consumption of fibre and fruit is associated with less coughing. They believe flavonoids are partly responsible.

American Journal of Respiratory and Critical Care Medicine, 2004

Action: Include the zest and juice of a lemon in your daily diet.

Bruises

These result from damage that makes blood leak from tiny blood vessels.

Lemon peel and juice may limit bruising and speed recovery because their flavonoids strengthen blood-vessel walls.

Action: Include the zest and juice of a lemon in your daily diet.

Cancer

Cancer results from mutation of a cell's DNA (genetic material). This produces malignant cells – meaning ones that continue multiplying instead of dying (from apoptosis – 'cell suicide') at their allotted time.

A lack of antioxidants encourages certain cancers. These normally mop up free radicals (unstable particles), which are continually produced in the body and can encourage cancer by damaging a cell's DNA.

Lemons – and especially their peel – contain almost every known type of cancer-preventing and cancer-fighting phyto-chemical, including carotenoids, flavonoids, limonene, pectin, glucaric acid salts, and terpenes.

Research suggests that:

- The flavonoid tangeretin helps prevent cancer growth by disturbing signalling between tumour cells.

- The flavonoid nobiletin can kill cancer cells, help prevent breast and colon cancers and certain leukaemias by inducing apoptosis of malignant cells, and make cancer cells less resistant to chemotherapy.

- The flavonoids naringenin and quercetin inhibit liver enzymes that convert the tobacco-related substance NNK into a potent inducer of lung cancer.

- Coumarins discourage cancer growth.

- Limonene helps prevent breast and colon cancers.

- Limonoids help fight cancers of the mouth, skin, lung, breast, stomach and colon.

- Glucaric acid salts discourage bowel cancer by promoting the production in the gut of butyric acid, which encourages apoptosis of malignant cells.

- Pectin's prebiotic properties help colon cells produce mucus, which helps stop carcinogens sticking to the gut lining.

- Pectin reduces the progression of advanced prostate cancer and makes mouth and throat cancers less likely to recur.

Researchers at the University of Arizona note that regular consumption of black tea containing lemon zest is associated with a reduction in skin-cancer risk of more than 70 per cent, black tea alone with a 40 per-cent reduction.

BMC Dermatology, 2001

A US study links a citrus-rich diet with a reduction in stomach cancer in men.

Cancer Epidemiology, Biomarkers & Prevention, 2001

Some alternative practitioners believe that our diet can influence cancer by affecting the metabolic processes that keep our body's pH (acid–alkaline) balance within its normal tightly controlled range. However, although cancerous tissue certainly may be unusually acidic, there is currently little evidence to support this view.

Action: Include the zest and juice of a lemon in your daily diet.

Cataracts

Clouding of the eye's lens affects many over-65s. Risk factors include diabetes, high blood pressure, smoking, infection and sunlight.

Studies suggest that the antioxidant power of vitamin C lowers the risk of cataracts by 80 per cent. Lemons are rich in antioxidants.

Action: Include the zest and juice of a lemon in your daily diet.

Cellulite

This dimpling of the skin is associated with excess tissue fluid and, perhaps, with unhealthy, inelastic collagen fibres tethering the skin.

Lemons can act as a diuretic, helping expel excess tissue fluid. They are also rich in vitamin C, which is needed for healthy collagen.

Action: Include the zest and juice of a lemon in your daily diet.

To boost circulation in affected areas, add 2 drops each of lemon and cypress oils to warm bath water, and rub your skin with a loofah.

Chapped lips

Lemon juice can be soothing.

Action: Stir a few drops of lemon juice into half a teaspoonful of Vaseline (petroleum jelly) or glycerine and smooth over your lips.

Chilblains

Lemon flavonoids can help the swelling and itching by reducing leakage of fluid from your capillaries (tiny blood vessels) into your skin.

Action: Include the juice and zest of a lemon in your daily diet.

Chronic illness

This can indicate a need for antioxidants such as vitamin C. Lemons are an excellent source and their flavonoids enhance the action of their vitamin C.

Lemon acids could help if you also have insufficient stomach acid and therefore poor absorption of certain nutrients. Low stomach acid affects one in two over-60s and can result from ageing, stress, the prolonged use of acid-suppressant medication, and an unhealthy diet high in meat, grain, sugar and carbonated drinks (which produce acid in the body) and low in vegetables and fruits. A lemon's acidity could aid digestion by lowering the pH of the stomach. Some alternative practitioners say, though without proof, that a deficiency of sodium from fruits and vegetables encourages the body to divert sodium from stomach-acid producing cells, so it's available to 'partner' acids in the urine and let them escape from the body. They say this could reduce the production of stomach acid.

Action: Include the zest and juice of a lemon in your daily diet.

Cold sores

The limonene in a lemon's juice and particularly in its oil has antiviral properties.

Lemon oil also helps by excluding air from a sore.

Action: Apply lemon juice to a cold sore several times a day, using a clean cotton pad each time.

Or add 1 drop of lemon oil to 2 teaspoons of sweet almond oil and apply this to the cold sore.

Colds, 'flu and sore throat

There is some scientific backing for the belief that taking at least 1g of vitamin C a day, starting from the first symptoms, reduces the likely length of a cold. However, it actually helps prevent colds only in people who undertake extreme exertion in cold weather (such as skiers). Also, since a lemon contains only around 60–100mg of vitamin C, you would need to consume a lot of lemons!

The flavonoids in lemons enhance the action of vitamin C. Also, some of them have anti-viral, anti-bacterial and anti-inflammatory properties. Quercetin, for example, has anti-viral properties.

The water in homemade lemonade helps replace fluid lost in sneezes, catarrh and – if you are feverish – sweat. Water makes catarrh moister and easier to shift, and helps prevent dehydration, which can cause headaches.

The decongestant vapour of lemon oil can shrink the swollen mucous membrane lining the air passages and Eustachian tubes. This eases breathing and discourages deafness.

Another benefit of lemons is that the bowel's bacteria ferment their pectin. This releases butyric acid and other short-chain fatty acids with prebiotic qualities – meaning they nourish 'good' probiotic bowel bacteria such as lactobacilli and bifidobacteria. These, in turn, benefit our immunity.

A German study of 479 volunteers found that taking tablets containing lactobacilli and bifidobacteria reduced the severity of colds, shortened their length by two days and increased the number of immune cells.

Clinical Nutition, 2005

Action: Drink 3–6 glasses of lemonade (see page 138) each day. Add two or three cloves or a small pinch of dried cinnamon to each glass to ease a fever.

Gargle with 1 teaspoon of lemon juice in a glass of warm water twice a day.

If you have gone deaf, put a few drops of lemon oil on a paper tissue and inhale its vapour.

Constipation

An unhealthy diet and dehydration are the likeliest causes.

Lemons are mildly laxative, partly because they are rich in pectin. This dissolves to form a gel in the bowel that makes stools softer and easier to pass. The cellulose in lemons also attracts water. This makes stools bulkier, softer and easier to pass, and reduces their transit time.

Action: Include the zest and juice of a lemon in your daily diet.

Corns and calluses

Ill-fitting footwear is usually to blame. Soaking the hard skin regularly in lemon juice and water, or lemon essential oil, should soften and hasten it's replacement with healthy skin.

Action: Add the juice of two lemons to a basin of warm water and soak your feet for 10 minutes a day. Then rub the softened skin away.

Alternatively, add 1 drop of lemon oil to 2 teaspoons of sweet almond or other carrier oil, rub the mixture into the hard skin and cover with cling film (plastic wrap) for 20 minutes. Repeat each day for a week.

Cough (*see also* Bronchitis)

Lemon essential oil is an expectorant, encouraging the airways to expel mucus.

A 5-year study of 63,257 people in Singapore suggests a diet high in fruit fibre discourages coughs.

American Journal of Respiratory and Critical Care Medicine, 2004

Action: Include the zest and juice of a lemon in your daily diet.

To soothe a cough:

- Drink homemade lemonade (see page 138).

- Put 2 tablespoons of cracked linseeds and half a lemon, sliced, into a pint of water, simmer for 20 minutes, then strain and sweeten with honey.

- Put 2 drops each of lemon essential oil, eucalyptus oil and tea-tree oil into a bowl of just-boiled water; put a towel over your head and inhale the vapour.

Cuts and grazes

A lemon's antiseptic properties can be useful.

Action: Gently clean the skin with a cotton pad soaked in lemon juice.

Dandruff

This flakiness is often associated with infection with the fungus *Malassezia furfur*. Lemon juice or oil may help.

Action: Apply a cup of lemon juice to the scalp, cover with a towel for 1 hour, then rinse and shampoo. Repeat once or twice a week.

Alternatively, if your scalp is dry, warm 2 teaspoons of coconut oil and mix with 1 drop each of lemon and chamomile essential oils. Massage your scalp with the mixture for 5 minutes, then cover with a hot towel for 20 minutes. Shampoo to remove.

Depression

The scent of lemon oil can affect mood, possibly via the brain's limbic system.

Backing for the suggestion that inhaling lemon-oil vapour can ease a depressed mood comes from researchers at Ohio State University.

Psychoneuroendocrinology, 2008

Action: Put a few drops of lemon essential oil into a diffuser or on a paper tissue and inhale the vapour every so often.

Diabetes

The raised blood sugar of pre-diabetes encourages diabetes, whilst untreated or poorly treated diabetes encourages heart, eye and kidney disease. Lemons might help in several ways.

Acid-containing foods seem very useful. Studies suggest that vinegar helps prevent high blood sugar. A lemon's acidity is similar to that of vinegar.

A study of 10 healthy volunteers at Lund University in Sweden found that adding vinegar to a breakfast of white bread reduced expected rises in blood sugar and insulin. This was attributed to the acid in the vinegar.

European Journal of Clinical Nutrition, 1998

Work at the same university found that eating pickled cucumbers with white bread and yoghurt dramatically lowered expected rises in blood sugar and insulin; fresh cucumbers did not.

American Society for Clinical Nutrition, 2001

In a study at Arizona State University, 21 people with pre-diabetes or diabetes drank water containing 2 tablespoons of vinegar before a carbohydrate breakfast. Doing this reduced insulin resistance by 34 per cent in those with pre-diabetes and 19 per cent in those with diabetes. The blood sugar was nearly 50 per cent lower in those with pre-diabetes, and 25 per cent lower in those with diabetes. Also, insulin levels improved.

Diabetes Care, 2004

A study of 12 healthy volunteers at Lund University found that taking vinegar with white bread increased satiety. The more vinegar, the greater the effect.

European Journal of Clinical Nutrition, 2005

In a study at Arizona State University, 11 people with diabetes consumed 2 tablespoons of vinegar and some cheese before bed-time. Their expected pre-breakfast blood-sugar level was reduced by 6 per cent next morning.

Journal of the Federation of American Societies
for Experimental Biology, 2007

All this suggests that vinegar reduces a meal's 'glycaemic index' (ability to raise blood sugar). Experts believe it delays stomach emptying, inactivates intestinal enzymes that convert complex sugars to glucose, and reduces the production and release of sugar from non-carbohydrate sources in the liver. Experts think that lemon juice, like other acidic foods, behaves in a similar way. Indeed, certain acidic foods have as powerful an effect on a meal's glycaemic index as the diabetes drug metformin. Frequent consumption of acidic foods is traditional in many countries and may help explain national variations in the rate of diabetes.

A lemon's fibre may help, too. 'Good' bowel bacteria break down pectin, liberating short-chain fatty acids, such as butyric acid, which reduce the release of sugar from the liver's stores. Short-chain fatty acids also inhibit C-reactive protein – a blood marker of inflammation and a predictor of diabetes.

Action: Include the zest and juice of a lemon in your daily diet.

Diarrhoea

Lemons might help in several ways.

Their pectin dissolves in the gut to form a gel. This helps bind the bowel contents into stools, which increases transit time. Also, 'good' gut bacteria break down some of the pectin. This forms a coating for the gut lining, which soothes irritation. It also releases butyric acid and other short-chain fatty acids with prebiotic qualities, meaning they nourish good ('probiotic') bowel bacteria such as lactobacilli and bifidobacteria. All this helps colon cells produce mucus, which helps prevent irritants sticking to and inflaming the gut lining. The cellulose in lemons attracts water in the bowel, making its contents more bulky and less runny.

Food acid, like stomach acid, helps kill diarrhoea-causing bacteria such as *Escherichia coli*. Lemons are particularly useful for people (such as one in two over-60s) with poor stomach-acid production. Indeed, certain West African villagers consume citric acid with a meal to protect themselves from cholera. The acidity of lemons (pH 2.1) is only a little less than that of stomach acid (pH 1–2).

The hesperidin that's concentrated in lemon pith may reduce bowel inflammation.

Journal of Pharmacy and Pharmacology, 1994

Action: Include the zest and juice of a lemon in your daily diet.

Fainting

Faints, or dizziness warning of them, can indicate that brain cells lack energy because the blood sugar is low.

The acidity and fibre content of lemons slows the absorption of sugar from the gut. This helps prevent blood sugar rising too high then dipping too low.

Lemon juice may particularly help those who lack stomach acid (such as one in two over-60s, and certain people who are stressed) and are also 'fast oxidizers' of sugar. Fast oxidizers quickly use up the readily available sugar in their blood, so feel hungry and, perhaps, faint soon after eating. Acidic foods, like stomach acid, promote protein digestion. This enables such people to get energy from protein, so they are less likely to faint.

Action: Include the zest and juice of a lemon in your daily diet.

Fatigue

Lemons supply small amounts of B vitamins, which can ease fatigue. Their fibre slows the absorption of sugar, which steadies blood-sugar levels and helps prevent low-blood-sugar dips, which can trigger fatigue.

Lemon acids could reduce tiredness associated with poor absorption of protein and certain other nutrients due to a lack of stomach acid. Low stomach acid is more likely with ageing, stress, prolonged use of acid-suppressant medication and a diet high in meat, grain, sugar and carbonated drinks (which produce acid in the body) but low in vegetables and fruits. A lemon's acidity could aid digestion by lowering the pH of the stomach. What's more, some alternative practitioners say, though without proof, that a deficiency in sodium from fuits and vegetables encourages the body to divert sodium from stomach-acid-producing cells so it's available to 'partner' acids in the urine. They say this could prevent the proper production of stomach acid. The sodium from lemons, though present in very small amounts, could help.

Research at Nagoya University in Japan found that giving rats acetic acid (as in vinegar) helped replenish sugar stores in their liver and muscle; this suggests that food acids in general may help prevent fatigue associated with low blood sugar.

Journal of Nutrition, 2001

London researchers have developed the ATP profile test, which indicates how well mitochondria (the cells' 'power-plants') are working. A study of 71 people with CFS/ME (chronic fatigue syndrome/ myalgic encephalomyelitis) and 53 healthy controls suggests that mitochondrial dysfunction causes fatigue.

International Journal of Clinical Experimental Medicine, 2009

US researchers believe that deficiencies of certain minerals and vitamins (including iron, zinc, magnesium, manganese, B vitamins – all present in small amounts in lemons) accelerate age-related mitochondrial decay.

Molecular Aspects of Medicine, 2005

Action: Include the zest and juice of a lemon in your daily diet.

Fibroids

One possible reason for these non-cancerous growths in the womb is an oestrogen/progesterone imbalance. This could activate genes that encourage womb-muscle fibres to proliferate. Another possibility is being very overweight, as fat cells produce oestrogen, and fat women tend to have high levels of blood sugar and growth hormone. A third possibility is pressure on and in the womb from congestion of blood and lymph in the pelvis.

The fibre in lemons reduces the numbers of gut bacteria that produce the enzyme beta-glucuronidase, which enables the reabsorption of oestrogen from the bowel into the blood. The B vitamins in lemons encourage the liver to break down surplus oestrogen. And their vitamin C – with help from flavonoids – strengthens tiny blood vessels (capillaries).

Action: Include the zest and juice of a lemon in your daily diet.

Fingertip splits

Splits in the skin at the ends of your fingertips are surprisingly painful.

Lemon essential oil can soothe the pain, soften the hard edges of cut skin and speed healing.

Action: Dig the fingertip into the under-surface of some lemon rind. This opens the lemon-oil glands and releases oil on to the split skin. Repeat two or three times a day until better.

Fishbone in throat

Lemon acids could soften a small fishbone and encourage it to be dislodged.

Action: Drink 1 tablespoon of lemon juice mixed with 1 tablespoon of olive oil every 2 hours for three doses. Eat some bread 1 hour after each dose.

Food intolerance

This can be associated with a lack of stomach acid (such as with stress, ageing, the unnecessary use of antacids or an unhealthy, acid-producing diet high in meat, grain, sugar and carbonated drinks but low in organic sodium from vegetables and fruits). Stomach acid enables the digestive enzyme pepsin to break down proteins; a shortage allows fragments of poorly digested protein to be absorbed into the blood, where they may trigger allergy.

A lemon's acids can mimic the action of stomach acid. Some practitioners say, though without proof, that the sodium in fruits and vegetables can help the body deal with an acid-producing diet by 'partnering' acids so they can escape in the urine. They say this means the body does not have to divert sodium from stomach-acid producing cells, which would prevent the proper production of stomach acid.

Action: If you suspect you lack stomach acid (for example, because indigestion is not eased by antacids), start each main meal with a salad dressed with lemon juice and olive oil, or a glass of water containing 2 teaspoons of lemon juice.

Fractures and sprains

Vitamin C aids collagen production, which means that getting sufficient vitamin C can help the healing of fractured bones of sprained ligaments.

Action: Include the juice of a lemon in your daily diet.

Gallstones

Most gallstones contain cholesterol; others contain bile pigments or calcium salts. Cholesterol-laden bile, and a poorly contracting gallbladder that can't expel small stones, are encouraged by obesity, constipation and diabetes. Bile can become unhealthily acidic, for example in people who eat an unhealthy diet, and stones are more likely to form in acidic bile.

A lemon's pectin helps bind bile acids in the gut, which prevents them from being reabsorbed and used to make gallstones.

Acidic foods such as lemon juice encourage the gallbladder to contract and expel bile and small stones.

A lack of stomach acid (as with ageing, stress, and medication with antacids or acid-suppressants) discourages gallbladder contractions, and stones readily form in stagnant bile. Lemon juice before a meal can mimic stomach acid.

Lemons as part of a healthy diet discourage any tendency of the body to become relatively more acidic. Lemons may also discourage acidity and gallstones, and certain practitioners suggest, though their suggestions are unproven, that their sodium may encourage the production of stomach acid.

A 'gallbladder flush' aims to soften stones and encourage gallbladder contractions. Very few success stories have been verified by X-ray or scan, and 'softened gallstones' reported in stools may just be lumps of soap made of bile salts and olive oil. But it may be worth trying.

Studies suggest that antioxidants discourage gallstones. Lemons are rich in antioxidants.

Cholesterol dissolves in limonene (albeit large amounts). Lemon peel contains limonene.

In one study, gallstones took 2 hours to dissolve in a test tube of limonene.

American Journal of Digestive Disease, 1976

In a study of 200 people, gallstones dissolved completely in 96, partially in 29, within 4 months of a limonene infusion into the gallbladder.

Digestive Diseases and Science, 1991

Action: Include the zest and juice of 1 or 2 lemons in your daily diet.

If you have stones, take 1 tablespoon each of lemon juice and olive oil 1 hour before breakfast each day.

Alternatively, consider a gallbladder flush (discussed first with a doctor). Drink 1 litre/35fl oz/4 cups of apple juice a day for 6 days. Next day, miss supper; at 9pm, take 1–2 tablespoons of Epsom salts in a little water; at 10pm, drink 4 tablespoons of lemon juice shaken with 125ml/4fl oz/½ cup of olive oil, then lie on your left side for 30 minutes before bedtime.

Gingivitis

Antioxidants and other anti-inflammatories in lemons may relieve the pain and swelling of unhealthy gums.

Action: Massage gums twice a day with lemon juice.

Alternatively, use an antiseptic and astringent mouthwash made with half water and half lemon juice, or with 1 drop of lemon essential oil in a cup of warm water.

Hay fever

Lemons might discourage hay fever and other allergic rhinitis because they contain anti-inflammatories and antihistamines, which may help prevent or ease an attack.

Action: Include the zest and juice of a lemon in your daily diet.

During an attack, consume 2 tablespoons of lemon juice in a glass of water three times a day.

If your throat is sore, gargle with 1 tablespoon of lemon juice in a cup of warm water.

Head lice

Lemon oil deters lice.

Action: Add 2 drops of lemon oil to your shampoo, and also add 2 drops to your conditioner or final rinse.

Headache

Some complementary practitioners believe headaches can result from our body's buffer systems working extra hard to keep the blood's pH (acidity–alkalinity level) within its normal, very slightly alkaline range of 7.35–7.45. Others believe that headaches can result from the blood's pH being at the higher (more alkaline) end of its normal range. They recommend treatment with vinegar. Interestingly, vinegar is a folk remedy familiar from the nursery rhyme in which Jack mends his head with 'vinegar and brown paper'. Lemon juice has similar acidity.

Action: Sponge your head with lemon juice, or apply a flannel (washcloth) soaked in 570ml/1 pint/2¼ cups of water containing 2 tablespoons of lemon juice.

Inhale mildly acidic vapour by putting 1 tablespoon of lemon juice into a vaporizer and staying close until it has evaporated. Alternatively, three times a day drink a cup of hot water containing 1 tablespoon of lemon juice.

Heart disease

The most common sort of heart disease – coronary artery disease – involves atherosclerosis, in which artery-lining (endothelial) cells leak, allowing penetration by lipids such as LDL-cholesterol and triglycerides. The lipids are then oxidized by free radicals, attracting white blood cells, which cause inflammation. Smooth-muscle cells produce collagen to cover leaks in the lining, and calcium infiltrates affected areas. All this stiffens blood vessels and prevents them from expanding and contracting as they should. It also forms plaques, which can rupture, causing clots that can trigger a heart attack. (Atherosclerosis can affect arteries elsewhere too; in the brain, for example, they encourage a stroke.)

Lemons can help many of the risk factors for coronary artery disease. They can reduce obesity, high blood pressure, diabetes, and high cholesterol, homocysteine (via their folate) and C-reactive protein (via their anti-inflammatories). Lemons can also reduce the oxidation associated with smoking and stress (via their antioxidants).

Researchers at Harvard University who monitored 76,283 women say the risk of heart disease was half in those who had 1 to 2 tablespoons of oil and vinegar dressing most days. They attributed this to the oil. But the vinegar may well have helped – and if so, lemon juice may be useful too.

American Journal of Clinical Nutrition, 1999

Studies suggest that flavonoids (as in lemon peel) discourage heart disease:

Finnish scientists who followed 5,133 people found the risk of heart-disease deaths was lowest in those who ate most foods rich in flavonoids.

British Medical Journal, 1996

A review by doctors at Boston University suggests flavonoids improve the behaviour of artery-lining cells and help prevent blood clots.

American Journal of Clinical Nutrition, 2005

'Good' micro-organisms in the bowel degrade pectin from lemons, freeing short-chain fatty acids such as butyric acid. These reduce LDL cholesterol, increase HDL cholesterol (the potentially protective sort) and inhibit C-reactive protein.

Researchers at Florida University found that giving pigs pectin reduced their expected arterial calcification.

Clinical Cardiology, 1988

Action: Include the zest and juice of a lemon in your daily diet.

Heavy periods

Possible triggers include stress, hormone imbalance, iron-deficiency anaemia, inelastic blood vessels due to a poor diet, fibroids, womb infection, and inflammation from a contra-ceptive device.

Lemon juice is a folk remedy. If it works, it's probably be-cause of some combination of its minerals (such as calcium, iron, magnesium and zinc), vitamins (such as beta-carotene and vitamin C) and flavonoids (such as rutin).

Action: Include the zest and juice of 2 lemons in your daily diet.

High blood pressure

Lemons can affect several of the risk factors, which include obesity, age, insulin resistance (pre-diabetes), salt sensitivity, and overactivity of the kidney hormone renin.

First, they encourage weight loss. Second, their potassium helps regulate body fluids, their magnesium relaxes arteries, their fibre encourages weight loss, their flavonoids promote arterial health and their acids discourage pre-diabetes.

In many people, fatty, chalky atheroma builds up in artery walls. Free radicals (encouraged by a poor diet, infection, smoking, stress) oxidize LDL cholesterol in atheroma, and trigger immune cells to inflame arteries. Atheroma and inflammation together stiffen the arteries, encouraging high blood pressure. Russian folklore recommends lemon and orange juice to help prevent this.

Studies suggest that hesperidin, a lemon flavonoid, reduces blood pressure in rats.

Journal of Nutrition Science and Vitaminology, 2003

Japanese researchers say that vinegar lowers blood pressure in rats. They think its acid reduces renin activity, which decreases angiotensin II, so decreasing blood volume and relaxing arteries. Lemon acids might act in a similar way.

Bioscience, Biotechnology, and Biochemistry, 2001

Third, lemons add flavour, encouraging people to add less salt.

Fourth, lemon juice releases calcium from meat or fish bones in casseroles or stocks; this could help those whose calcium intake is low, since calcium promotes healthy blood pressure.

Fifth, vitamin C in lemons can boost nitric oxide, which relaxes blood vessels.

Sixth, lemon juice resembles ACE-inhibitor medication as it inhibits angiotensin-I-converting enzyme (ACE); this decreases production of the hormone angiotensin, which raises blood pressure by constricting blood vessels.

When rats with high blood pressure consumed lemon juice, their blood pressure tended to fall. The Japanese researchers attributed this to inhibition of ACE by flavonoids such as hesperidin and eriocitrin.

Food Science and Technology International Tokyo, 1998

Action: Include the zest and juice of a lemon in your daily diet.

High cholesterol

An unhealthy diet and insufficient exercise and sunlight encourage too much LDL (low density lipoprotein) cholesterol in the blood, plus too little HDL (high density lipoprotein) cholesterol, and high levels of total cholesterol and triglycerides (types of fats now properly called triacylglycerols). The liver makes 80 per cent of the body's cholesterol from triglycerides and a substance called apolipoprotein B. Various constituents of lemons can influence this production.

Oxidation of LDL cholesterol by free radicals (enhanced by stress, sunlight, exercise and smoking) encourages high blood pressure, heart attacks and strokes. The vitamin C, phenolic compounds (including flavonoids), pectin, limonin and acids in lemons encourage healthy cholesterol levels.

Citrus flavonoids reduce LDL cholesterol in hamsters, probably by reducing production in the liver.

Journal of Agricultural and Food Chemistry, 2004

Pectin thickens the bowel contents, which reduces the absorption of cholesterol from food and bile and helps eliminate it. Also, 'good' gut bacteria degrade pectin, liberating short-chain fatty acids such as butyric acid, which inhibit cholesterol absorption, suppress its production in the liver, and boost HDL cholesterol.

Studies show that pectin plus vitamin C lowers cholesterol more than pectin alone, and pectin plus phenolic compounds lower cholesterol and triglycerides more than either alone.

Lemons are richer than apples in pectin. Eating one large apple each day lowers cholesterol by up to 11 per cent; two lower it by up to 16 per cent; and four have the cholesterol-lowering power of a statin drug!

Researchers at Florida University found that giving pectin to pigs reduced cholesterol by 30 per cent and reduced expected arterial calcification.

Clinical Cardiology, 1988

The US Agricultural Research Service found that liver cells produce less of the protein apo B (needed to make LDL cholesterol) when exposed to limonin.

Journal of Agricultural and Food Chemistry, 2007

Alternative practitioners claim that a healthy diet containing plenty of 'alkaline-forming' foods, such as lemons, helps dissolve and eliminate cholesterol.

Research suggests that a lemon's glucaric acid salts reduce LDL cholesterol by up to 35 per cent.

Nutrition Research, 1996

Action: Include the zest and juice of 1 or 2 lemons in your daily diet.

Indigestion and heartburn

Lemon juice makes fried food more digestible because its acids emulsify ('cut') fats so that they don't lie on the stomach, and aid protein digestion – which is particularly useful for the many people who lack sufficient stomach acid, such as one in two over-60s, and those who are stressed or take antacids unnecessarily. Also, lemons are metabolized to potassium carbonate, which helps reduce any excess acidity in the body. Finally, limonene may help prevent heartburn (perhaps by coating the gullet lining and thus protecting it from acid) and promote healthy stomach movements.

A study of 19 adults found that taking 1,000mg of limonene every day or two relieved heartburn and acid reflux.

U.S. Patent (642045), 2002

Action: Include the zest and juice of a lemon in your daily diet.

For heartburn, drink 1 tablespoon of lemon juice in a glass of warm water.

Infection

Lemon oil has some degree of antibacterial, antiviral and anti-fungal action, mainly thanks to its limonene and antioxidants. The flavonoid hesperidin may help prevent serious infection.

Action: Include the zest and juice of a lemon in your daily diet.

Infertility

Vitamins B, C and E, folic acid, selenium and zinc in lemons help nourish sperm and eggs and help sperm swim.

Action: Include the zest and juice of a lemon in your daily diet.

Insomnia

Inhaling the vapour of lemon oil is said to have sedative properties.

Action: Add a few drops of lemon essential oil to your bath water.

Alternatively, massage your stomach with a few drops each of lemon, ylang ylang (antidepressant, confidence-boosting) and vetivert (sedative, comforting) essential oils. Lie down, put a few drops of the mixture on your palm, relax and move your hand around the outer margin of your abdomen in smooth, slow, clockwise circles.

Another option is to put a few drops of lemon oil on your pillow at bedtime.

Irritable bowel syndrome (IBS)

Possible symptoms include pain, constipation, diarrhoea, passing mucus, bowels never feeling empty, wind and bloating. One in three people sometimes has an irritable bowel; one in five of these has frequent trouble, known as irritable bowel syndrome.

The pectin in lemons may reduce symptoms by making stools softer and easier to pass.

Action: Include the zest and juice of a lemon in your daily diet.

Itching

Lemon juice is said to reduce itching.

Action: Bathe in tepid bath water containing the juice of 2 lemons.

Alternatively, apply lemon juice to itchy skin.

Kidney stones

Stones are more likely to form if you have an unhealthy diet. Lemons can help prevent stones by providing calcium, magnesium, selenium, vitamin B and fibre.

In particular, consuming lemon juice may help dissolve stones that contain uric acid or calcium. Calcium-containing stones are more likely to form when threatened over-acidity of body fluids leads to calcium being withdrawn from bones and teeth and excreted in the urine to help keep the pH (acid–alkaline balance) of body fluids within its normal range. The metabolism of the acids in lemon juice has a mild alkalinizing effect in the body, so consuming lemon juice could help prevent this type of stone.

Stones are also more likely in people with pre-diabetes, as their raised blood sugar level after eating carbohydrate raises insulin, which, in turn, makes their kidneys discharge calcium in the urine. A lemon's acidity discourages high blood sugar.

Action: Include the zest and juice of a lemon in your daily diet.

To reduce pain from a stone, drink the juice of half a lemon in a glass of water every half an hour for 4 hours or until the pain subsides.

Low immunity

Lemons contain vitamin C, which boosts immunity. In addition, their pectin fibre is degraded by 'good' micro-organisms in the large bowel, liberating short-chain fatty acids, such as butyric acid. These aid immunity by stimulating the production of helper T cells, antibodies, white blood cells and cyto- kines. They also inhibit C-reactive protein, which is a marker of inflammation.

Action: Include the zest and juice of a lemon in your daily diet.

Macular degeneration

Vitamin C in food discourages age-related macular degeneration (AMD, deterioration of 'straight-ahead' sight), say Dutch researchers. They followed up 4,170 over-55s for about eight years, and found that the 560 who developed AMD ate less vitamin-C-rich food than the others. Supplements of vitamin C made no difference.

Action: Include the zest and juice of a lemon in your daily diet.

Memory loss

Lemons are rich in antioxidants, and studies of mice suggest these discourage memory loss.

Action: Include the zest and juice of a lemon in your daily diet.

Metabolic syndrome

This is some combination (subject to debate) of high fasting blood glucose levels (pre-diabetes), high blood pressure, an apple-shaped body, low HDL cholesterol and high triglycerides. It encourages diabetes, heart disease and strokes, affects one in five people, and is also known as insulin resistance syndrome or syndrome X. It's more likely with increasing age and can be associated with polycystic ovary syndrome. Most sufferers are sedentary, obese and insulin-resistant. Researchers suspect that inflammation and oxidation play a part. Certainly, affected people are more likely to have a high level of C-reactive protein, indicating inflammation.

Lemon antioxidants and acids may help to prevent pre-diabetes, high blood pressure, obesity and unhealthy levels of cholesterol and triglycerides.

Action: Include the zest and juice of a lemon in your daily diet.

Miscarriage

Studies suggest that antioxidants make miscarriage less likely.

Action: Include the zest and juice of a lemon in your daily diet.

Mouth ulcers

Lemon oil is reputed to ease the pain of aphthous ulcers.

Action: Mix 3 drops of lemon, 3 of tea tree and 2 of myrrh essential oils with 1 tablespoon of sweet almond or other carrier oil. Apply a few drops to the ulcer with your finger every 2 hours.

Or apply lemon juice several times a day.

Muscle stiffness

Pain and stiffness experienced after exercise might respond to anti-inflammatories such as nobiletin in lemon oil.

Action: Put 1 teaspoon of lemon oil in your bathwater and relax for half an hour.

Alternatively, add 3 drops of lemon oil and a few drops of ginger oil (an analgesic and local circulation booster) to 3 tablespoons of sweet almond or other carrier oil, and massage the muscles with the mixture.

Neuralgia

The cooling and anti-inflammatory properties of lemon juice may ease pain from an irritated nerve.

Action: Apply warmed lemon juice over the painful area and repeat each hour for half a day.

Alternatively, add 3 drops of lemon oil to 2 tablespoons of sweet almond or other carrier oil, and smooth over the affected area. Or add a few drops of lemon oil to the water in an aroma-therapy diffuser, or put them in a bowl of just-boiled water and lean over it with a towel over your head, to inhale the vapour.

Nosebleed

Lemon juice has astringent properties, and a lemon's peel, pith and core are rich in rutin and other flavonoids that can strengthen blood vessels.

Action: Soak a cotton ball in lemon juice, lean your head

backwards, then put the ball in the affected nostril and leave for 10 minutes.

If you have frequent nosebleeds, include the zest and juice of a lemon in your daily diet.

Obesity

Lemons contain pectin, which forms a gel in the digestive tract. This mops up triglyceride fats and reduces their absorption; it also increases satiety.

Researchers in Texas found that pectin increased satiety.
Journal of the American College of Nutrition, 1997

Lemon acids and pectin slow the absorption of sugar after a meal with a high glycaemic index (blood-sugar-raising effect), which in turn slows the rise in blood sugar. This helps prevent low blood-sugar dips, which can trigger overeating.

Research suggests that food acids promote weight loss. Vinegar, for example, aids satiety and speeds the burning of calories. It also helps compensate for any lack of stomach acid. The latter affects one in two over-60s, and is encouraged by stress, the prolonged use of antacid or acid-suppressant medication, and an unhealthy, acid-producing diet such as one rich in meat, grain, sugars and carbonated drinks but low in fruits and vegetables. A lack of stomach acid is associated with the poor absorption of many nutrients, which encourages overeating. Vinegar improves nutrient absorption by increasing the stomach's acidity. Also, by improving protein digestion, it may help people who are 'fast oxidizers' of sugar and therefore feel hungry soon after a meal. This is because it enables them to produce energy from protein when they have used up the readily available blood sugar. Lemon juice has similar acidity to vinegar, so should be equally beneficial.

Women in their 50s gained 2.25kg/5lb less over 10 years when they took calcium supplements. This suggests many were previously short of calcium – possibly because they lacked stomach acid, as in 40 per cent of women of this age. Taking vinegar with meals would improve their calcium absorption.

On-line report from the Fred Hutchinson Cancer Research Center, Seattle, 2006

The sodium in fruits and vegetables may help prevent a lack of stomach acid due to an acid-producing diet. This is because it can 'partner' acids so that they can escape in the urine. This means that the body does not have to divert sodium from stomach-acid-producing cells. This is good news because sodium is vital for the production of stomach acid.

The vitamin C in lemons could aid weight loss, too, as the following study suggest.

Studies at Arizona State University found that volunteers with adequate vitamin C burnt 30 per cent more fat during exercise than those with low levels. Also, when obese women who were trying to lose weight took vitamin C, they lost twice as much. We need adequate vitamin C to produce enough carnitine – an amino acid that helps our body burn fat well.

American College of Nutrition, 2005

Action: Include the zest and juice of a lemon in your daily diet. If the stomach produces too little stomach acid, calcium is absorbed in an insoluble form, which means it cannot be ionized and absorbed in the bowel.

Osteoporosis

Affected bone is light and fragile. Risk factors include a lack of 'bone-friendly' nutrients, such as calcium, magnesium, zinc and vitamin C. Lemons help provide these.

Researchers suspect that inflammation may play a part in osteoporosis; lemons provide anti-inflammatories such as nobiletin. Other risk factors for osteoporosis include age, too much exercise and smoking. These encourage oxidation by free radicals, which research increasingly suggests may be an underlying factor. Lemons contain a wide variety of antioxidants.

Hesperidin decreases bone density loss in mice.
Journal of Nutrition, 2003

Lemon pectin may be useful, too, because gut bacteria break it down, releasing short-chain fatty acids (such as butyric acid), which raise acidity in the large bowel. This boosts the absorption of bone-friendly minerals such as calcium and magnesium.

Lemons as part of a healthy diet help prevent any tendency of the blood to be at the lower (and hence relatively more acidic) end of the normal range of pH (acid–alkaline balance – the normal range being 7.35–7.45). This is because lemons are metabolized in the body to produce alkaline end-products. This helps prevent the need for the body to take calcium and other minerals from the bones in order to accompany and thus get rid of acid in the urine. A diet rich in meat, grain, sugars and carbonated soft drinks encourages a tendency to increased acidity in the blood; a diet rich in vegetables and fruits such as lemons discourages it.

Finally, lemon acids provide acidity in the stomach for those who lack enough for good calcium absorption. A lack of stomach acid can reduce calcium absorption by 80 per cent. It affects one in two over-60s and is more common in people who are stressed, habitually take antacids or acid-suppressants, or eat an acid-producing diet high in meat, grain, sugar and carbonated drinks and low in fruit and vegetables. A lemon's sodium can help the body deal with such a diet by 'partnering' acids so that they can escape in the urine. This means the body does not have to divert sodium from stomach-acid producing cells, and in so doing prevent the proper production of stomach acid.

Action: Include the zest and juice of a lemon in your daily diet.

Peptic ulcer

An ulcer can develop if something interferes with the stomach's protective mucus, lining cells or acid. Unfortunately, many people lack stomach acid, including one in two over-60s and many of those who are stressed, are habituated to antacids or acid suppressants, or eat an acid-producing diet rich in meat, grain, sugars and carbonated drinks and low in fruits and vegetables. Inflammation from infection with *Helicobacter pylori* bacteria is a major cause of stomach ulcers, inflammation (gastritis) and cancer. Around two in five of us are infected, though only one in 10 infected people get an ulcer. It's a common misconception that people with ulcers make too much acid. In fact, most don't, and many make too little.

Japanese research indicates a strong correlation between low stomach acidity and increased rates of *H. pylori* infection.

Biotechnic and Histochemistry, 2001

It's possible that if someone with peptic ulcer symptoms tests positive for *H. pylori* and suspects a lack of stomach acid (for example, because antacids don't relieve their symptoms), the acidity of lemon juice might discourage the infection.

Also, a lemon's sodium can help the body deal with an acid-producing diet by 'partnering' acids so that they can escape in the urine. This means the body does not have to divert sodium from stomach-acid producing cells to do this. This is good, because sodium is necessary for stomach-acid production.

Action: Drink a glass of water containing 2 teaspoons of lemon juice with each meal, or add lemon juice to some of your everyday recipes.

Piles

Piles are spongy pads in the walls of the anus (back passage) that have become bulky and loose. They readily become inflamed, and inflammation can cause discomfort, itching and bleeding. Causes include constipation and fragile veins. Lemons can help, as their vitamin C and rutin and certain other flavonoids strengthen veins; their fibre helps prevent constipation; and their anti-inflammatory antioxidants reduce inflammation.

Action: Include the zest and juice of a lemon in your daily diet.

Pre-eclampsia

Studies suggest that antioxidants lower the risk of this pregnancy problem, which can cause high blood pressure, protein in the urine and ankle swelling. Lemons contain a wide variety of antioxidants.

Action: Include the zest and juice of a lemon in your daily diet.

Pre-menstrual syndrome

Pre-menstrual syndrome is probably caused by changes in levels of neurotransmitters, such as serotonin and GABA (gamma-amino butyric acid), resulting from oversensitivity to the changing balance of progesterone and oestrogen during this part of the menstrual cycle. Research suggests that glucaric acid salts help by suppressing the enzyme beta-glucuronidase. This enables a process called glucuronidation in the liver, which makes oestrogen more water-soluble and thus aids its elimination in the urine.

Limonene also encourages glucuronidation.

Action: Include the zest and juice of a lemon in your daily diet during the 2 weeks before you expect a period.

Prolapse

Among the many possible causes of a 'sagging' womb are straining due to constipation, a chronic cough and weak pelvic muscles and ligaments.

Lemons may help prevent a prolapse, or stop it getting worse. This is because they can help cure constipation or a cough, and their vitamin C and rutin and certain other flavonoids promote healthy muscles and ligaments.

Action: Include a liquidized lemon in your daily diet several times a week.

Psoriasis

Patches of thick flaking skin overlie inflammation on the knees, elbows, scalp or elsewhere.

Citric acid in lemon juice can ease dryness and flaking. In addition, the sun's ultraviolet-A rays act on psoralens in lemon juice to mimic the PUVA (psoralen-UVA) therapy used for psoriasis by dermatologists.

The anti-inflammatory effects of a lemon's carotenoids and certain flavonoids (such as hesperidin) may soothe inflammation.

Action: Smooth lemon juice over psoriasis several times a day.

Treat patches with juice, as above, then expose them to sunlight for a few minutes a day, increasing the time over several weeks. Include the zest and juice of a lemon in your daily diet.

Restlessness

Lemons might help, as they contain the flavonoid hesperidin.

Hesperidin can act as a sedative, possibly via action on the body's opioid or adenosine receptors.

European Journal of Pharmacology, 2008

Action: Include the zest and juice of a lemon in your daily diet.

Scurvy

This results from a lack of vitamin C and causes fatigue, bleeding gums, easy bruising, dry flaky skin, poor healing and thin hair. It used to be a problem for sailors on long voyages, so ships were required to carry enough lemon or lime juice for each sailor to have 25g/1oz a day after 10 days at sea.

Lemon juice is one of the best sources of vitamin C, and the flavonoids in lemons aid its beneficial actions.

Action: Include the juice of a lemon in your daily diet.

Stress

The body's need for certain nutrients – including vitamins B and C, calcium, magnesium, potassium and zinc – rises during stress. Lemons can help with their supply.

In addition, the scent of lemon oil is said to alleviate stress.

Action: Include the zest and juice of a lemon in your daily diet.

Consider using a few drops of lemon essential oil in an aromatherapy diffuser or massage blend.

Strokes

A stroke ('brain attack') usually results from a blood clot interrupting the blood flow in one of the brain's arteries (when it's called a thrombotic stroke). Less often it's caused by bleeding in the brain from an unhealthy artery (a haemorrhagic stroke). The main culprits behind a thrombotic stroke are the narrowing, roughening and inflammation of an artery in the brain by atheroma (see Heart disease). Clots readily form in affected arteries, especially if there are also other risk factors, such as smoking, stress, an unhealthy diet, obesity, high blood pressure, diabetes and chronic infection.

Lemons can help many of the risk factors for strokes. They can help reduce obesity, high blood pressure, diabetes and high cholesterol, homocysteine (via their folate) and C-reactive protein (via their anti-inflammatories). Lemons can also reduce the oxidation associated with smoking and stress (via their anti-oxidants).

The vitamin C and flavonoids in lemons may discourage several possible causes of strokes. Research suggests that flavonoids in lemon peel help prevent oxidation of LDL cholesterol. Flavonoids are also thought to reduce cholesterol production in the liver.

A review by doctors at Boston University suggests flavonoids improve the behaviour of artery-lining cells and help prevent blood clots.

American Journal of Clinical Nutrition, 2005

'Good' micro-organisms in the bowel degrade pectin from lemons, freeing short-chain fatty acids such as butyric acid. These reduce LDL cholesterol, increase HDL cholesterol (the potentially protective sort) and inhibit C-reactive protein.

Researchers at Florida University found that giving pigs pectin reduced their expected arterial calcification.

Clinical Cardiology, 1988

Action: Include the zest and juice of a lemon in your daily diet.

Sunburn

The antioxidants in lemons could discourage sunburn.

Action: Include the zest and juice of a lemon in your daily diet.

Mix 3 drops of lemon oil into 2 tablespoons of sweet almond or other carrier oil and apply this to your skin.

Alternatively, apply lemon juice.

Urine infection

If infection is making your urinary tract inflamed and sore, overly acidic urine – for example, from an unhealthy diet – will worsen the pain. The urine's normal pH (acid–alkaline balance) varies from 4.5 to 9, the ideal perhaps being 5.8 to 6.8. The metabolism of lemon juice in the body has a mildly alkalizing effect that can help restore your urine to its normal state.

Action: Consume the juice of half a lemon 2 or 3 times a day.

Varicose veins

Lemons can act as a venous tonic as they have strengthening, astringent and anti-inflammatory effects on vein walls.

Action: Include the zest and juice of a lemon in your daily diet.

Massage your legs with a mixture of 2 drops of lemon, 2 of lavender and 3 of cypress essential oils in 2 tablespoons of sweet almond or other carrier oil.

Warts

Both lemon juice and lemon oil are reputed to help cure warts.

Action: Consume the juice of half a lemon twice a day at least.

Apply 1 drop of lemon essential oil to your wart and cover with a sticking plaster. Repeat each day for 2 weeks.

CHAPTER FOUR

Beauty Aid

Every part of a lemon contains beautifying ingredients. Lemon juice can cleanse, soften and moisturize your skin, condition and lighten your hair and deodorize your body. Lemon oil is moisturizing and toning. It also has a light, fresh, appealing fragrance that can lift the spirits, and when diluted with a carrier oil it is lovely for a massage. Another reason why lemon juice is such a good beauty aid is that its organic acids can help maintain or restore the skin's natural acidity.

Normal skin has a slightly acidic surface layer called the acid mantle or hydro-lipid film. This contains:

- the fats (lipids) of skin oil (sebum)

- the lactic acid and amino acids of sweat

- the amino acids and pyrrolidine carboxylic acid of dead skin cells

The skin's normal pH (acid/alkaline balance) over most of the body in women is 4.5–5.75 (below 7 on this scale is acidic, above is alkaline). Men's skin is slightly more acidic.

This slight acidity helps repair damaged skin and activates enzymes that enable the production of lipids in sebum. This helps explain why water finds it hard to escape from the skin (other than in perspiration) and harmful substances and micro-organisms find it hard to enter. It also encourages healthy populations of bacteria and fungi on the skin and helps prevent infection. Reduced acidity – caused, for example, by most soaps, and by eczema or other dermatitis – encourages drying, cracking and itching.

Most soaps, even mild, glycerine or baby ones and beauty bars, have an alkaline pH of 7–9, which temporarily destroys the skin's normal acidity. In healthy skin, the acidity generally recovers between 30 minutes and two hours (or more), though twice-daily soaping compromises this degree of restoration. Certain soaps are particularly alkaline (pH 9.5–11). The pH of Dove soap is relatively low at 6.5–7.5, but only a very few bar soaps (for example, Cetaphil and Aquaderm) have a pH similar to that of normal skin. However, the pH of many liquid soaps, non-soap cleansers and bath and shower gels resembles that of normal skin more closely; and the pH of a few (for example, Johnsons pH 5.5 Hand Wash) is similar to that of normal skin.

Using a cleanser containing lemon juice avoids any reduction in acidity. Or, if you want to use alkaline soap, you can rinse your skin afterwards with a 'splash' of diluted lemon juice.

Lemon acids are moisturizing. This is partly because they help maintain or restore the skin's acidity, which helps prevent water loss, and partly because a lemon's citric acid is an alpha-hydroxy acid (AHA, used in many commercial skin-care preparations), meaning it has an intrinsic moisturizing action. It also loosens dead skin cells and encourages them to flake off. So it can soften and smooth rough or hard skin and help cracked skin to heal.

The softening produced by citric acid helps explain why applying lemon juice makes blackheads easier to remove with gentle fingertip pressure or a blackhead extractor. What's more, the astringent properties of lemon juice tend to contract large pores, so there's less space for blackheads in them. Also, the vitamin C and other antioxidants in lemon juice help prevent lipids in sebum from being oxidized and therefore blackened by air to create a blackhead.

Rutin and certain other flavonoids in lemons can strengthen the walls of the capillaries, our tiniest blood vessels. So including the zest and juice of a lemon in your daily diet could help prevent the tiny broken veins that sometimes occur on the face and elsewhere.

The moisturizing and softening properties of its acids make lemon juice an excellent aid for a manicure or pedicure.

Caution: Avoid putting neat lemon oil on your skin within 12 hours before sunlight exposure. Or use no more than one drop per 2 teaspoons of sweet almond or other carrier oil, so it's unlikely to trigger a photosensitive reaction.

Diluted lemon juice also restores acidity to just-washed hair. Most shampoos are alkaline, so they temporarily destroy the scalp's normal acidity, leaving it prone to dryness, irritation and even infection. Their residues also dull the hair. A lemon rinse not only makes hair shine but can also enhance natural highlights.

Cleansing

- Steam-clean your face by putting 900ml/30fl oz/3¾ cups of just-boiled water into a bowl and adding the full-thickness peel of half a lemon, 1 teaspoon of dried mint (or 2 of chopped fresh mint), 1 teaspoon of dried parsley (or 2 of chopped fresh parsley) and, for dry skin, the contents of a capsule of evening primrose oil. Sit for 5 minutes with your face over the bowl and a towel over both your head and the bowl. Then rinse with lukewarm water.

Exfoliating

- Get rid of dead cells by rubbing damp skin with lemon-scented salt in a warm bath. Make it by putting 225g/8oz/¾ cup of sea-salt (of the type used in a salt grinder) into a bowl and stirring in half a teaspoon of lemon essential oil. Keep the mixture in a screw-top jar.

Toning

- Mix the juice of a lemon with twice its volume of water, and refrigerate in a covered container. After cleansing your face, apply some of this lemon toner with a cotton pad and leave to dry.

Moisturizing

- Smooth lemon juice over your skin, wait for half an hour, then rinse. Or, to soften hard elbows, sit with each one in a squeezed-out half-lemon shell for the same length of time.

Smoothing fine lines and wrinkles

- Lemon juice is a valuable part of this facial mask. Stir a well-beaten egg white together with 1 teaspoon of egg yolk, 1 tablespoon of lemon juice and a drop of vitamin E oil from a capsule. Apply to your face, then lie down for half an hour. Wash and dry your skin and apply some moisturizer.

Blackheads

- Smooth lemon juice over the affected skin and let it dry. Repeat each day as necessary.

Deodorizing

- Because it has anti-bacterial properties, lemon juice can act as a deodorant. Rub the cut surface of a lemon over each armpit or simply add the juice of a lemon to your bath water.

Broken veins

- Consume the zest and juice of a lemon each day to provide your veins with strengthening rutin and other flavonoids.

Massage

- Lemon oil blends well with many other essential oils, including lavender, rose, neroli, sandalwood, geranium and ylang ylang, for a soothing massage oil.

Manicure or pedicure

- Soften cuticles and whiten stained hands and nails by soaking them for 10 minutes in a bowl of warm water containing the juice of half a lemon. Gently push back your cuticles. Then rub a strip of lemon peel on your nails to make them shine.

Hair care

- After shampooing greasy hair, rinse with water plus a squeeze of lemon juice. Its acidity counteracts dullness by reducing the alkalinity of traces of shampoo. It also dissolves soap residues that were in the shampoo, which in turn releases fatty acids. All this gives hair an attractive shine and texture.

- Similarly, after shampooing dry hair, rinse with water plus a squeeze of lemon juice. Like many commercial dry-hair-care products, this contains an organic acid (citric acid), which chelates ('binds') unwanted traces of heavy metals and shampoo that can further dry the hair.

- After bleaching or colouring your hair, rinse with water containing a squeeze of lemon juice. Lemon acids precipitate proteins, which helps counteract hair damage caused by the bleach or colouring agent.

- Lemon juice can give your hair a sun-kissed effect. Rinse clean wet hair with 185ml/6fl oz/¾ cup of water mixed with 4 tablespoons of lemon juice. Sit in the sun until your hair dries.

CHAPTER FIVE

Household Help

Lemons are useful for many household chores and can help keep your home fresh, clean and sparkling. Note that it is fine to use bottled lemon juice instead of fresh lemon juice for household tasks.

Air-freshening

- Half-fill the bowl of a ceramic diffuser with water, add a few drops of lemon essential oil (*Citrus limonum*) and light the nightlight (tea light). The vapour of the oil is said to help lift the spirits, clear the mind and improve concentration.

- Add a few drops of lemon essential oil to a spray bottle half-filled with water, shake well and spray to make the air in a room smell fragrant.

- Leave thinly pared strips of lemon peel to dry out well over several days, then put them in your wardrobe or chest of drawers to scent your clothes.

- Add strips of dried lemon peel to a bowl of fragrant dried flowers or leaves for a *pot pourri* to scent a room. Sprinkle the contents of the bowl every couple of weeks with a few drops of lemon essential oil to refresh the aroma.

- Make a wonderfully scented pomander by studding a lemon with cloves, then tying some ribbon around it so you can hang it up.

- Deodorize the drain of your kitchen sink by putting the juice of a lemon into a glass of water and pouring the lemon water down the plughole.

- Remove the odour of fish, onion or garlic from your hands by rubbing them with fresh lemon juice.

- Freshen your vacuum-cleaner bag by sprinkling a few drops of lemon essential oil on to a paper tissue and putting this into the bag.

- Keep your fridge smelling sweet by putting half a lemon on a saucer.

- Make your air humidifier smell good by adding a few drops of lemon juice to its water container.

- Make a waste-disposal (garbage disposal) unit smell fresh by putting the peel of a lemon through it and rinsing with water.

- To freshen a carpet or rug, mix 10 drops each of lemon and lavender essential oils into 125g/4½oz/1 cup of bicarbonate of soda (baking soda). Put in a covered container over-night so the bicarbonate of soda absorbs the oil. Next day, sprinkle the mixture over the carpet or rug, then vacuum up the powder.

Cleaning

- Use lemon essential oil to clean kitchen and bathroom surfaces, as its limonene is a solvent that removes greasy marks as well as alcohol does.

- Remove grease with lemon juice.

- For a cleaner for wooden, laminate or ceramic-tiled floors, pour into a spray bottle 240ml/8fl oz/1 cup of white vinegar, 240ml/8fl oz/1 cup of water, 5 drops of lemon essential oil, 2 drops of tea tree essential oil and 5 drops of lavender essential oil. Spray this mixture on to the floor and wipe clean with a microfibre cloth or a mop. Alternatively, add 4 tablespoons of white vinegar and 10 drops of lemon essential oil to a bucket of water and mop the floor with this scented solution.

- To clean and deodorize a microwave cooker, mix 30g/1oz/¼ cup of baking soda, 1 teaspoon of vinegar and 6 drops of lemon essential oil together. Use a sponge to apply this paste to the inside of the microwave. Rinse with water and leave the door open for 15 minutes to allow for drying.

- To remove limescale from around a plughole or tap, rub with the cut end of half a lemon, then rinse.

- To clean windows, rub the cut surfaces of a lemon quarter over the glass, wipe off with a damp cloth, then dry with a dry cloth.

Polishing

- Use lemon essential oil to polish surfaces, as its limonene acts as a solvent, dissolving old wax, fingerprints and grime.

- Brighten copper cookware or ornaments by dipping half a lemon into salt, bicarbonate of soda (baking soda) or baking powder, then rubbing it over the surface. The lemon acids dissolve the tarnish, and the salt, bicarbonate of soda or baking powder act as a mild abrasive to clear it away. Rinse with water and dry with a cloth or a paper towel.

- To make a furniture polish, combine in a glass jar 2 parts olive oil with 1 part strained fresh lemon juice. This polish accentuates the beauty of the wood; it also nourishes it and prevents it from drying out.

- Polish dulled surfaces of aluminium or chrome objects by rubbing with the cut surface of half a lemon, then buffing with a cloth.

Disinfecting

- Add a squeeze of lemon juice to disinfect drinking water that you think might be contaminated with bacteria.

- Use lemon essential oil to clean kitchen, bathroom and other surfaces that are likely to be contaminated with bacteria. Several of its constituents, including limonene, have anti-bacterial properties.

- Disinfect kitchen chopping boards with lemon juice, as it contains citric and other acids, and bacteria dislike an acidic environment.

Stain removing

- If your hands are stained (for example, after peeling onions), rub them with lemon juice to remove the stains.

- To remove sweat stains from clothes, scrub gently with half and half lemon juice and water.

- To remove stains from white laundry, mix 1 tablespoon each of lemon juice and cream of tartar and apply the mixture to the stain. Leave for a few minutes, then rinse with water. For persistent or extensive staining on a fabric that is washable in very hot water, boil the item in a pan containing 5 tablespoons of cream of tartar to every 1.1 litre/2 pints/4½ cups of water, then rinse.

- For stains on fabrics that can be washed in hot water, pour 240ml/8fl oz/1 cup of lemon juice into the washing machine during the wash cycle.

- An alternative method is to dampen the stain and sprinkle it with cream of tartar. Carefully hold the stained area in the steam from a boiling kettle, then rinse well with water.

- To remove rust spots or mildew stains on washable clothing, sprinkle the area generously with salt, then squeeze fresh lemon juice over it. Leave the item for several hours, ideally in direct sunlight. Keep the stain moist by applying more lemon juice as necessary. Brush off the salt and then launder as usual. (Be warned – putting household bleach on rust spots will set the stain.)

- Sprinkle lemon juice over berry stains on clothing or other fabric, to help them fade.

- Mix 1 tablespoon of bicarbonate of soda (baking soda) with a few drops of fresh lemon juice to form a paste, then rub this over stains on plastic food-storage containers.

- Leave fresh lemon juice for 45 minutes on stains on Formica worktops. Then sprinkle with bicarbonate of soda (baking soda), scrub gently and rinse.

Dealing with insects

- If kitchen or other cupboards are infested with insects, wipe them with lemon essential oil on a cloth. Its limonene is toxic to insects but not to humans.

- Use a rotten lemon to repel ants.

- Put strips of dried lemon peel into a little muslin bag and place in cupboards and drawers to repel clothes moths.

- Sprinkle lemon juice around door thresholds and on windowsills, as its scent will deter the entry of insects.

CHAPTER SIX

Choosing and Using Lemons

Several tips are worth knowing before buying lemons and when storing and using them at home.

Choosing lemons

Ideally, choose lemons that are fresh, healthy and full of juice. Such a lemon will look good, smell good and taste good. It will also provide plenty of juice and a firm rind, as well as nutrients and other health-promoting substances.

When selecting a lemon, check that it:

- Feels firm, full and heavy but has some 'give' when you press it – avoid one that is hard and shrivelled (as it be may be old and desiccated) or soft and squidgy (as it may be decaying).

- Is well shaped and free from scabs or streaks, spots or other discoloration, which could be associated with viral, bacterial or fungal infection or damage during harvesting and post-harvest washing and storage.

- Is free from scars, which could have been caused by burning or other injury from pesticide sprays or fumigation.

- Is free from pitted or sunken areas on the rind, which could have resulted from excessive oil-spraying before harvest, or excessive chilling, mechanical brushing or humidity afterwards.

- Has bright, shiny yellow peel, which shows it is well ripened; a greenish or pale yellow lemon is more acidic.

- Has a uniform colour, which indicates that the peel is not infected and the lemon has been well handled.

- Has unbroken peel, since a break could have enabled intrusion by infecting micro-organisms.

- Ideally has a coarsely 'pebbled' rind, which indicates that it's likely to keep well.

- Has rough, thick peel if you particularly want its zest, as the yield will be greater.

- Has thin, smooth peel if you particularly want its juice, as the yield will be greater.

- Is unwaxed if you want to use its zest or rind, as it will be free from the wax, fungicide and other substances that are sprayed on lemons during commercial storage. Such lemons are sometimes sold as 'organic'.

When you cut open a lemon, check that it is juicy. Dryness shows that it has been kept too long or is unhealthy. Check too that its pith and membranes are whitish and its pulp pale yellow, since discoloration can be sign of a fungal infection (for example, red, brown or black staining suggests infection with the black-rot fungus, *Alternaria*, that is most likely to affect trees in wet weather). Discoloration can also result from damage by excessive chilling after a lemon has been harvested.

Storing lemons

You can store a lemon for three weeks, perhaps longer, in a sealed plastic bag or a tightly lidded jar in the refrigerator, or for one to two weeks at room temperature and out of direct sunlight. You can keep lemon juice in an airtight container in the refrigerator for up to five days. Alternatively, you can put juice into ice-cube trays and freeze them for use at a later date. Lemon zest can be stored in an airtight container in a cool dry place, or put in an airtight freezer bag and frozen. You can also put small strips of lemon zest in water into ice-cube-tray compartments so you can enjoy the look and taste of lemon in ice for drinks.

Lemon slices or wedges (see pages 90–91) can be pre-prepared and kept in a plastic bag in the refrigerator for three or four days.

Washing lemons

If a lemon is waxed, then before grating or cutting its rind for use in drinks or food, or before liquidizing it whole, gently brush or rub it with hot water and washing-up liquid for one minute, then rinse it well in plain water. This is sensible because most lemons are sprayed after harvest with an aqueous emulsion of wax (such as carnauba wax) plus a pesticide to prevent them drying out and help avoid infection. Alternatively, dip the lemon in just-boiled water for half a minute to dissolve the wax, then remove the lemon and brush it under running water.

Using lemons

Lemon wedges

There are several ways to prepare lemon wedges ('quarters') to accompany fish or other dishes so the user won't get sprayed with juice when squeezing the juice from the wedge. First, cut the lemon in half lengthways, then cut each half into two or three wedges, depending on the size of the lemon. Next, choose one of the following:

- Best of all, cut a tiny piece from the two pointed ends of the wedge with a sharp knife, then use sharp scissors to cut off any of the lemon's central white core, and to dig out the pips.

- Wrap the wedge in a circle of muslin, secured by knotting its free edges or binding them with fine string; while this looks wonderful, you may think it over the top.

- Give each diner a little hinged lemon press (available from cook shops).

Lemon slices

To prepare lemon slices, cut the lemon in half crossways, then cut slices crossways from each half.

To prepare notched-edge slices, take a lemon slice and cut notches in its peel.

To prepare lemon twists as a garnish for food or drinks, take a lemon slice, cut it from its centre to its edge, then twist each cut end in opposite directions. Secure with a cocktail stick if using for a drink.

Lemon zest

There are various ways to remove the zest, depending on the result you want:

- For finely grated zest, use a metal grater, taking care to move the lemon frequently, and not to grate your fingers! (Use a stiff pastry brush to remove the zest from the grater.)

- For very fine 'julienne' strips, use a citrus zester.

- For wider strips, use a vegetable paring knife or a vegetable peeler, cutting the zest either down the length of the lemon or in one continuous spiral strip around the lemon; cut the strips with a sharp knife to make them thinner, if necessary.

- For yellow-stained zesty sugar, rub the zest off with sugar lumps, then use them in recipes.

Note that when grating zest for decoration, grate only the yellow part, not the white pith beneath too, as this is particularly bitter. However, when producing zest to include in a healthy diet, or for medicinal reasons, it's fine to include some grated pith, as its flavonoids and other phenolic compounds are good for us.

Always remove the zest from a lemon before removing its

juice. If you don't need it immediately, you can then store it (see page 89) for use later in various recipes.

Lemon juice

To get the maximum volume of juice from a lemon, it needs to be at room temperature. If it has been kept in a fridge, remove it a couple of hours before juicing it. Alternatively, put it in a bowl and cover with just-boiled water for half a minute. Next, roll the lemon with your hand on a flat surface, as this helps to release the juice by breaking down the lemon's internal membranes.

Finally, squeeze out the juice using one of the following:

- Your hands.

- A citrus reamer (a plastic, wooden, metal or ceramic ribbed rounded-cone-shaped device that you twist into the lemon).

- A citrus trumpet (a metal gadget that you screw into the lemon, then squeeze the lemon juice by hand into it).

- A lemon squeezer (a glass, ceramic or metal ribbed device with a pip catcher and a juice-collecting area).

- An electric lemon squeezer.

You can add the leftover lemon pulp to the juice if you want.

Note that bottled lemon juice is available, which can be handy if you get caught short, but it does not taste nearly as good as fresh juice. One reason is that the contents of bottled juice are slightly different from those of fresh juice: for example, there is less vitamin C in bottled juice. Another reason is that it's likely to contain preservatives, such as sodium benzoate or sodium metabisulfite. (It's worth noting here that sodium metabisulfite can trigger an allergic reaction in certain people.) On the plus side, though, bottled juice is usually cheaper than fresh juice, and it also lasts longer, so you may like to use it in home-made cleaning products (see Chapter 5).

Invisible ink

You can amuse children by showing them how to make invisible ink. Simply mix the juice of a lemon with a few drops of water in a small bowl. Then use a cotton bud to write on white paper with this 'ink'. As the ink dries, it should become virtually invisible. To reveal the writing, carefully hold the paper near a light bulb. As the lemon juice heats up, it is oxidized by the air, which darkens it and reveals the writing.

Lemon lore

- Note that one medium lemon yields 2–3 tablespoons of juice, 2 teaspoons of grated zest and 7–10 slices.

- Use lemons as soon as possible after cutting them.

- If you have cut a lemon, used part of it and want to store the remainder, either cover the cut surface in clingfilm (plastic wrap) or coat it in vinegar (if it is going to be used in something savoury).

- Brush lemon juice over the cut surfaces of bananas, apples, pears, peaches and avocados that you need to keep for a while, as this keeps their colour by preventing oxidation. Similarly, dip cut white vegetables (such as potatoes or parsnips) in a bowl containing a cupful of water mixed with 1 tablespoon of lemon juice.

- Add a few drops of lemon juice to an electric juicer to help prevent fruit or vegetable juice going brown.

- Add a few drops of lemon juice to whipping cream if it doesn't whip.

- Use a little lemon juice or grated zest instead of salt in recipes, to reduce your intake of sodium.

- Add lemon juice when cooking cauliflower or green vegetables, to brighten their colour.

- Ease peeling of the shells of hard-boiled eggs by adding a squeeze of lemon juice to the water before boiling them.

- When boiling eggs, help prevent their shells cracking by adding a squeeze of lemon juice to the water in the pan.

- When a recipe for cooked food contains lemon juice, add the juice after cooking if possible, as heating increases the loss of vitamin C.

- Add lemon juice when cooking rice, to make it fluffier.

- Intensify the flavour of mushrooms by adding lemon juice when you cook them.

- Add lemon juice when cooking fish, as lemon acids prevent unwanted fishy cooking odours by neutralizing substances called amines in the flesh.

- Make the skin of a roast chicken or duck extra crispy by rubbing it with lemon juice before cooking it.

- Revive a limp lettuce by putting it in a bowl of cold water containing the juice of half a lemon then putting the bowl in the refrigerator for an hour.

Lemon alert

Be wary of accepting lemon slices in drinks in restaurants and pubs, since they could make you unwell unless prepared with scrupulous hygiene. The background to this is a study in New Jersey in which researchers ordered drinks containing lemon slices at 21 restaurants. Tests showed that 77 per cent of the lemon slices contained staphylococci, Shigella (dysentery bacteria), or other infectious organisms. This probably means that the restaurant employees either handled the lemons without first washing their hands with anti-bacterial soap (a severe violation of the health code in most US states – indeed, in Alabama, for example, employees must wear gloves, or use tongs or deli sheets), or that they cut raw meat, then used the unwashed knife to cut the lemons.

CHAPTER SEVEN

Recipes

The wonderful shiny, sunlit yellow of a lemon brings bling to your kitchen, while the popular flavour of its juice and peel add a fresh, tart zing to all kinds of recipes, from starters through to vegetables, fish, poultry, meat, desserts, cakes, breads, drinks and many other foods.

Please note:

- Each recipe serves 4.

- 1 tsp (teaspoon) = 5ml; 1 tbsp (tablespoon) = 15ml; 1 cup = 240ml/8fl oz

- All fruit and vegetables are medium-sized unless otherwise stated. When medium lemons, which yield about 2 tbsp juice, are unavailable, use small (which yield about 1 tbsp) or large (3–6 tbsp) lemons as necessary.

- Use unwaxed lemons when possible, especially if the zest is to be used in a recipe. If using unwaxed lemons, wash them first (see page 89)

- All egg are medium (US large) unless otherwise stated.

- If you are using a fan oven, reduce the temperature recommended in the recipe by 20ºC/25ºF.

- Salt is included only when necessary for curing or softening other ingredients. This is because some people prefer to avoid added salt, and anyone who wants to can easily add it at the table.

Starters (Appetizers)

Many lemon-containing starters come from Middle Eastern and Mediterranean countries, where lemons are produced and used in abundance. Avgolemono (egg and lemon soup) and slices of halloumi cheese fried with lemon are two of the best-loved recipes. Pasta coated with lemony, buttery breadcrumbs is a family favourite that is perhaps the ultimate in comfort food and nowadays graces tables far beyond Italy, its mother country. Finally, taramosalata (lemon-flavoured fish roe dip), salmon mousse and sardine-stuffed lemons are three examples of how brilliantly lemons complement fish.

AVGOLEMONO

This creamy-textured Greek soup offers a magical combination of flavours. Any tiny pasta shapes are suitable, including con-chiglietti (shells), farfalline (bows), orzo ('rice'), stellette (stars) and filini (threads). Ideally, use stock made by boiling a chicken carcass in water for 1 hour with onions, carrots, celery, a splash of vinegar (to release calcium from the bones) and herbs.

> 1.75l/3 pints/7¼ cups chicken stock
> 100g/3½oz/½ cup small pasta shapes
> 3 eggs
> juice of 1½ lemons (remaining ½ lemon sliced)
> black pepper
> 4 tbsp fresh parsley, chopped

Bring the stock to the boil and cook the pasta in it for 5 minutes, or for as long as instructed on the packet.

Break the eggs into a bowl and whisk until frothy. Stir in the lemon juice plus 2 tablespoons of the hot stock. Slowly pour this mixture into the pan, stirring well. Reheat gently, without boiling, as this would make the eggs curdle. Season with pepper.

Divide the soup between 4 bowls, sprinkle with parsley and garnish with the slices of lemon.

HALLOUMI WITH LEMON

Originating in Cyprus and popular in Greece and the Middle East, this firm, almost rubbery cheese is made from goats', sheeps' and, sometimes, cows' milk. It absorbs other flavours well, and, rather than melting when cooked, it remains intact and develops a golden crust.

200g/8oz halloumi, thinly sliced
juice and grated zest of 1 lemon
3 tbsp olive oil
4 tsp fresh or 2 tsp dried oregano or marjoram

Lay the halloumi slices in a shallow dish. Put the zest of the lemon, the juice of half the lemon and the olive oil in a bowl, mix well and pour over the cheese. Cover and leave to marinate in the refrigerator for 4–12 hours.

Remove the cheese slices from the marinade and fry for 1–2 minutes on each side in a nonstick pan until golden-brown. Put the slices on a plate, pour the remaining marinade over them, and sprinkle with oregano or marjoram. Serve with good bread and salad leaves.

PASTA WITH LEMON AND BREADCRUMBS

Pasta with breadcrumbs (*pasta con il pangrattato*) is a very popular Italian dish, and lemon juice and zest can make it extra special. Fettuccine holds the coating well, but any pasta is suitable. To ring the changes, you might like to substitute cream for the second half of the olive oil, or stir in some tinned anchovies.

    325g/12oz fettuccine, spaghetti or tagliatelle
    6 tbsp olive oil
    25g/1oz/2 tbsp butter
    3 garlic cloves, crushed
    2 slices of day-old bread, made into breadcrumbs
    juice and grated zest of 1 lemon
    handful of fresh parsley, chopped
    black pepper

Cook the pasta according to the instructions on the packet.

Meanwhile, heat half the oil, and the butter, in a large nonstick pan, add the garlic and cook for 30 seconds, stirring. Add the breadcrumbs and cook, stirring often, for a further 5 minutes or until lightly browned.

Drain the pasta and put it in a bowl. Stir in the lemon juice and zest, then the breadcrumbs and parsley, and season with plenty of black pepper.

TARAMOSALATA

This Greek dip is made from hard roe (fish eggs). Its name comes from preserved carp or grey mullet roe ('tarama'), but carp is usually used in Greece now, and cod, salmon or white-fish roe is fine too. The roe can be smoked; salted ('cured'); or salted, pressed and dried. Carp roe is light pink (from natural carotenoid pigments) or darker pink (from added colouring); mullet roe is amber; and cod roe is whitish. You can buy pre-served roe from certain fishmongers or in cans from Greek food shops, certain supermarkets or on-line. If using salted roe, soak it in cold water for two hours first, to remove some of the salt.

    2–3 slices of bread, crusts removed
    100g/3½oz plain or smoked cod or carp roe
    240ml/8fl oz/1 cup olive oil
    juice of 2 lemons
    black olives or fresh parsley or basil leaves, to garnish

Soak the bread in water, then squeeze dry. Put the bread and roe into a food processor or blender and blend until mixed. Add the oil and lemon juice slowly, then pulse until creamy and thick. (Use a little warm water to dilute if it gets too thick.) Put in the refrigerator to chill.

Garnish with black olives or some herbs and serve with wedges of lemon and either pitta or slices of crusty bread.

SALMON MOUSSE

This tangy salmon starter is always warmly received. It looks attractive when turned out from a ring mould, but it tastes just as good from any other tin or dish.

juice of 2 lemons (to make 6 tbsp)
1 sachet (12.5g/½oz) powdered gelatine (unflavoured powdered gelatin)
1 tbsp caster (superfine) sugar
1 tsp mustard
425g/15½oz tinned salmon, drained
2 celery sticks, finely diced
1 tbsp capers
150ml/5fl oz/scant ⅔ cup double (heavy) cream, whipped to soft peaks
1 cucumber, peeled and finely sliced
1 small bunch of watercress
1 lemon, quartered

Put the lemon juice and 6 tablespoons of cold water into a large bowl and sprinkle the gelatine on top. Stand the bowl carefully over a pan of boiling water and stir until the gelatine dissolves. Stir in the sugar and mustard, remove the bowl from the pan and leave to cool.

Remove any soft bones from the salmon then stir it in to the bowl with the celery, capers and cream. Pour the mixture into an oiled ring mould and refrigerate for at least 6 hours.

Run a basin of very hot water and carefully immerse the mould (taking care not to wet the mousse) for a few seconds. Remove it from the water. Run the point of a knife around the inner and outer edges of the mousse. Put a serving plate over the mould, turn both upside-down, and gently dislodge the mousse on to the plate.

Garnish with cucumber around the base and watercress in the centre, and lemon quarters for squeezing.

SARDINE-STUFFED LEMONS

This recipe was particularly popular in the 1970s, but it's quick and easy to prepare and its appearance and flavour certainly justify a place on our tables today.

4 lemons
1 can sardines in oil
25g/1oz/2 tbsp butter
2 spring onions (scallions), finely chopped
1 celery stick, finely chopped
2 tbsp mayonnaise
pinch of black pepper
a few sprigs of fresh parsley

Cut off the tops of the lemons, scoop out the pulp and discard it. Cut the bottom from each lemon so it will stand upright. Drain the oil from the can of sardines into a saucepan, add the butter and spring onions and cook, stirring, for 5 minutes. Remove from the heat and let it cool.

Mash the sardines and add to the pan with the celery, mayonnaise and pepper. Stir and use the mixture to stuff the lemon shells. Replace the lemon tops, inserting a few sprigs of parsley so they stick out from each gap. Serve with thin slices of wholemeal toast.

Vegetables and Salads

A squeeze of lemon juice into the cooking pan can lend piquancy to many a vegetable, including green leaves, roots, peas and beans.

SPINACH WITH LEMON

The flavours of lemon juice and onion make lightly cooked spinach even more of a treat. Note that squeezing the washed spinach really well, so that relatively little water seeps from it as it cooks, helps retain its goodness.

    1 onion, finely sliced
    3 tbsp olive oil
    1 kg/2lb fresh spinach, washed, torn up and squeezed
    black pepper
    ½ lemon

Put the onion and olive oil into a large frying pan and fry gently for 10 minutes. Add the spinach and pepper and stir well. Cover and cook gently for 7 minutes. Add the juice of the lemon and serve hot or cold.

ROOT AND SEED SALAD WITH LEMON

This colourful raw-vegetable salad is a delightful surprise to many people.

4 small beetroot, peeled and grated
4 carrots, peeled and grated
handful of fresh parsley, chopped
handful of fresh mint, chopped
juice of 2 lemons
2 tbsp olive oil
50g/2oz/½ cup sunflower seeds
50g/2oz/½ cup pumpkin seeds

Put the beetroot, carrots and herbs into a large bowl with the lemon juice and oil.

Heat a large frying pan and dry-fry the sunflower and pumpkin seeds for 5 minutes, tossing frequently, until golden and toasted.

Add the seeds to the bowl and toss the ingredients together.

LEMON (NIMBU) DAL

Dal, meaning 'split pulses cooked with spices and vegetables', is popular in India, Nepal, Pakistan and Bangladesh, where it is often eaten with rice or flat breads. Options include masoor dal (red lentils), urad dal (black lentils), toor dal (yellow pigeon peas), chana dal (chickpeas) and mung dal (mung beans). This recipe is for lemon-flavoured masoor dal.

225g/8oz/1 cup dried red lentils, rinsed
1 large potato, cut into quarters
3 tbsp olive oil
1 tsp ground cumin seeds
1 tbsp ground coriander seeds
½ tsp ground fenugreek seeds
½ tsp ground turmeric
½ tsp ground cinnamon
½ tsp ground cloves
¼ tsp ground chilli
½ tsp ground black pepper
2 onions, finely sliced
2 garlic cloves, crushed
2.5cm/1in fresh root ginger, chopped
2 tomatoes, chopped
1 tbsp grated coconut
juice and grated zest of 1 lemon

Put the lentils and potato into a saucepan with plenty of water. Bring to the boil and simmer for 15 minutes or until the potato is tender. Remove the potato. Continue cooking the lentils for a further 10 minutes or until tender (the cooking time of a pulse depends on its type and age). Drain them, then put them back in the pan, add the potato and mash them together.

Heat the oil in a large heavy-based frying pan. Add all the dried spices and the black pepper and fry, stirring, over a high heat for 1 minute. Then add the onions, garlic and ginger, and cook over a lower heat for 10 minutes or until the onions are soft. Add the tomatoes and cook for another 5 minutes or until they are pulpy, then add the coconut, lemon juice and zest. Finally, add the mashed lentil and potato mixture, and stir – adding a little water if necessary – until heated through.

LEMON ROAST POTATOES

Potatoes roasted with lemon juice and butter are an excellent option for accompanying a Sunday roast of pork or lamb.

    1 kg/2lb potatoes, peeled and cut into large chunks
    juice of 1 lemon
    75g/3oz/6 tbsp butter
    black pepper
    handful of fresh parsley, chopped

Preheat the oven to 190°C/375°F/gas 5.

Put the potatoes into a roasting tin, sprinkle with the lemon juice, dot with the butter and season with the pepper. Pour 150ml/5fl oz/scant ⅔ cup hot water into the tin.

Cook in the oven for 1 hour 5 minutes, basting twice, and adding a little water if necessary. Turn the temperature up to 200°C/400°F/gas 6 and cook for another 15 minutes. Sprinkle with parsley before serving.

Fish, Shellfish, Poultry and Meat

It's common knowledge that adding lemon juice to cooked fish and shellfish makes them even more delicious, but it's also well worth using lemons when preparing and cooking seafood. For example, lemon juice enhances the flavour of salmon as it cures and of herring as it cooks. As a marinade it 'cooks' raw fish (by altering its protein structure) and gives it a lovely lemony tang at the same time.

Lemons also go really well with chicken and other meats, as with a lamb tagine or stuffed cabbage or vine leaves. And you're in for a treat if you slip some halved lemon shells around a sizzling roasting chicken or piece of pork, because heat softens them and mellows their flavour in a most attractive way.

GRAVAD LAX WITH LEMON AND DILL

Dry-curing with salt is an ancient way of preserving salmon, trout, herring and other oily fish. Sugar and dill enhance the flavour of the salmon in the popular Scandinavian recipe for gravad lax. Adding lemon zest at the same time gives an even more lemony flavour than just squeezing lemon juice over the fish before you eat it. Once prepared, gravad lax keeps in the refrigerator for at least five days.

    1 kg/2lb 4oz salmon fillet with skin
    3 tbsp sea salt (preferably flakes)
    2 tbsp caster (superfine) sugar
    2 tbsp coarse-ground pepper
    grated zest of 2 lemons, plus 1 lemon cut into quarters
    bunch of fresh dill, chopped, or 2 tbsp dried dill

Check the salmon fillet with your fingertips and pull out any small remaining bones with tweezers. Cut the fillet across its length into two halves.

Cut a piece of foil large enough to wrap around the salmon and lay it in a dish.

Mix the salt, sugar, pepper and lemon zest in a bowl, and sprinkle a quarter of the mixture over the foil-lined base of the dish.

Lay one half of the salmon fillet, skin-side down, on the foil and sprinkle a third of the remaining salt mixture over the top. Lay the fresh dill (reserving a few sprigs for decoration) or scatter the dried dill over the fish, and sprinkle with half the remaining salt mixture.

Place the other half of the fillet, skin-side up, over the first. Cover with the remaining salt mixture, then wrap the foil loosely over the top. Put a baking tray over the wrapped fish, weight it down with several tins of food or other heavy items, and refrigerate for 24 hours.

Unwrap the fish and turn it over, then spoon the juices over the top. Re-wrap the fish and refrigerate for another 12–24 hours.

Unwrap the fish, wash off the salt mixture under running cold water and pat dry with kitchen paper. Cut into thin slices and decorate with the reserved dill sprigs and the lemon quarters. Serve with salad leaves, and sour cream or mayonnaise.

TUNA CEVICHE

A marinade of lemon or lime juice 'cooks' raw fish, making it tender and pale, because the fruit acids break down the long protein molecules. Ceviche is a traditional South American dish.

> 900g/2lb fillets of tuna, or sole or other white fish, skin removed, cut into strips
> 1 red onion, finely sliced
> 2.5cm/1in fresh root ginger, grated
> juice and grated zest of 6 lemons
> 1 tsp sugar
> 1 tsp cumin seeds, toasted and ground
> 5 tbsp olive oil
> black pepper
> 2 avocados, peeled, pitted and sliced
> ¼ watermelon, peeled, deseeded and cubed
> 300g/11oz peeled cooked prawns (shrimp)
> handful of coriander (cilantro) leaves

Put the strips of fish, half the onion slices, the grated ginger and the juice of 5 of the lemons into a bowl and mix gently. Cover and refrigerate for 2 hours, spooning the juices over the fish every 30 minutes.

Put the remaining onion slices and lemon juice into a non-metallic bowl with the sugar and ground cumin, and leave for half an hour, mixing several times.

To make the dressing, drain the liquid from around the marinated onions into another bowl and mix with the oil and lemon zest, then season with black pepper to taste.

Discard the liquid and onion slices from around the marinated fish. Now stir in the marinated onion slices, avocado slices, watermelon cubes, prawns and dressing.

Decorate with coriander (cilantro) leaves.

LEMON-SOUSED HERRINGS

Sousing herring fillets in lemony or vinegary water and baking them in the oven is a quick and easy way to prepare this delightful supper dish.

8 small herrings, filleted
1 onion, finely sliced
8 peppercorns
4 bay leaves
juice of 4 or 5 lemons (to give 180ml/6fl oz/¾ cup juice)

Preheat the oven to 180°C/350°F/gas 4.

Roll up the herring fillets and secure each with a wooden cocktail stick. Put the rolled herrings into a shallow oiled ovenproof dish and add the onion, peppercorns and bay leaves. Pour the lemon juice over the herrings and add the same amount of water, just to cover them.

Cover with foil and bake for 45–60 minutes, until tender. Drain and serve hot with mashed potatoes. Alternatively, cool in the cooking liquid, drain and serve as a starter.

ROAST CHICKEN WITH LEMON AND THYME

Roast chicken with lemon and thyme plus lots of garlic scents your home with the most wonderful aromas and is an almost universally popular 'comfort food'. If your chicken is of a different weight from the one in the recipe below, cook for 20 minutes per 500g/1lb 2oz, plus an extra 20 minutes.

75g/3oz/6 tbsp butter, at room temperature
juice and grated zest of 1 lemon (empty lemon halves retained)
4 tsp fresh or 2 tsp dried thyme
1 tbsp quince or crab-apple jelly (or redcurrant jelly)
large pinch of black pepper
1 chicken weighing roughly 1.6kg/3lb 8oz
5 bay leaves
2 garlic bulbs, halved across
3 tbsp olive oil
120ml/4fl oz/½ cup boiling hot chicken stock

Preheat the oven to 180°C/350°F/gas 4.

Put the butter into a bowl and mix in the juice and zest of the lemon along with the thyme, quince or crab-apple jelly, and pepper. Loosen the skin away from the chicken breasts, then stuff three-quarters of the butter mixture beneath the skin.

Put the chicken into a greased roasting tin and smear the remaining butter mixture on its upper surface. Put the bay leaves and garlic bulbs around the chicken and sprinkle with the olive oil. Cook for 30 minutes.

Remove from the oven and pour the stock around the chicken. Slice the empty lemon halves and scatter close to the chicken. Cover the pan with foil, and cook for 60 minutes. Remove the foil and cook for 15–20 minutes more, or until the juices run clear when you stick a skewer into a fleshy part of the chicken. Use the pan juices to make gravy by adding to the roasting tin a little boiling water or cooking water from steamed or boiled vegetables.

CITRUS AND SAGE PORK CHOPS

This easy-to-prepare dish looks colourful and festive, the pork has a welcome succulence and tartness and many people find the roasted citrus shells surprisingly moreish.

  1 onion, chopped
  4 pork loin chops
  3 garlic cloves, crushed
  2 tbsp fresh sage, chopped, or 1 tbsp dried sage
  2 tsp honey
  juice of 2 lemons (retain the empty lemon halves)
  juice of 2 oranges (retain the empty orange halves)
  3 tbsp balsamic vinegar
  2 tbsp olive oil
  1 tbsp fresh parsley, chopped

Preheat the oven to 230°C/450°F/gas 8.

Put the onion into a roasting tin and lay the pork chops on top. Mix the garlic, sage, honey, lemon and orange juice, balsamic vinegar and olive oil together and pour over the chops. Place alternating lemon and orange shells around the chops.

Reduce the oven temperature to 180°C/350°F/gas 4 before putting the pork in, then roast for about 30 minutes. Serve with the juices poured over the top.

LAMB TAGINE

Named after the earthenware pot with a conical lid traditionally used in Morocco and other North African countries, this
colourful stew has a fragrance that is redolent with herbs and
the mellow scent of preserved lemon.

800g/1lb 12oz boneless shoulder of lamb, cubed

4 garlic cloves, crushed

small handful of fresh parsley, chopped

small handful of coriander (cilantro) leaves, chopped, but leaving
   a few whole

½ tsp ground cinnamon

1 tsp ground cumin

1 tsp paprika

pinch of black pepper

4 tbsp olive oil

2 onions, finely chopped

1 sweet potato, peeled and cubed

2 carrots, peeled and cut into sticks

2 red bell peppers, deseeded and sliced

225g/8oz/1¼ cups dried (preferably unsulphured) apricots

2.5cm/1in fresh root ginger, grated

240ml/8fl oz/1 cup passata, or 5 tomatoes, finely chopped

240ml/8fl oz/1 cup vegetable or lamb stock

1 preserved lemon, rinsed, and sliced if necessary

50g/2oz flaked (slivered) almonds

juice and grated zest of 1 lemon

Preheat the oven to 180°C/350°F/gas 4.

Put the lamb into a large ovenproof casserole that can also go on the hob. Mix the garlic, parsley, coriander, cinnamon, cumin, paprika, black pepper and oil in a jug and pour over the lamb. Cover with clingfilm (plastic wrap) and leave to marinate in the refrigerator for at least 4 hours.

Cook the casserole over a high heat for 5 minutes, stirring, then add the onions, sweet potato, carrots, red peppers, apricots, ginger, passata and stock, and bring to the boil. Transfer to a tagine if you have one, or cover the casserole, and put it in the oven for 2 hours.

Stir the preserved lemon and flaked almonds into the casserole and cook for a further 5 minutes. Stir in the lemon juice and sprinkle with the zest and reserved coriander leaves. Serve with couscous or rice.

STUFFED CABBAGE LEAVES WITH EGG AND LEMON SAUCE

'Dolmathes' is Greek for 'stuffed vegetables', and stuffed cabbage leaves are just one example, others include stuffed vine (grape) leaves, aubergines (eggplant), courgettes (zucchini), bell peppers and tomatoes.

    1 large green cabbage
    450g/1lb minced (ground) lamb or pork
    2 tbsp olive oil
    100g/3½oz long-grain rice, soaked for 30 minutes then rinsed
        and strained
    2 onions, finely sliced
    3 tbsp fresh flat-leaf parsley, chopped
    1 tbsp fresh dill, chopped
    pinch of black pepper
    3 eggs, separated
    50g/2oz/4 tbsp butter
    2 small lemons
    2 tbsp cornflour (cornstarch)

Cut the leaves from the cabbage, working from the outside in, removing the core and the lower part of the thick central vein of each leaf. Wash the leaves, and soften them by immersing a few at a time in boiling water for 1–2 minutes, then draining. Retain the largest leaves for lining the saucepan (see below). Cut the largest few of the remaining leaves in half, to use as wrapppers.

Put the lamb, oil, rice, onions, parsley, dill and pepper into a bowl. Beat 2 of the egg whites (the third white is not used) and stir them into the mixture. Put 1 tablespoon of the stuffing on each leaf and each halved large leaf, and wrap the leaf around to secure the stuffing and form a fairly tight package.

Line a large saucepan with the retained large outer leaves, then pack in the stuffed leaves, placing a few knobs of butter in between each layer. Put an inverted plate over the top layer. Pour in enough hot water to cover the stuffed leaves, cover and bring to the boil, then simmer for 50 minutes.

Press on the plate, and drain the liquid from the saucepan into a bowl and make up to at least 150ml/5fl oz/scant ⅔ cup with water. Set aside.

Put the 3 egg yolks into a small bowl and beat with a fork. Add the lemon juice and beat again. Put the cornflour into another small bowl, stir in 2 tablespoons of water, then beat into the egg mixture. Now add the liquid retained from the pan of stuffed cabbage, 1 tablespoon at a time and beating constantly until you have added 4–5 tablespoons. Pour over the stuffed leaves in the pan, then return the pan to the heat and reheat for 3–4 minutes, rotating the pan occasionally.

Desserts

The tartness of lemons and the sweetness of sugar marry exceptionally well, which explains why there are so many popular recipes for lemon-flavoured desserts. Some excellent ones that I've had to leave out are pancakes with lemon and sugar, lemony rice pudding, lemon cheesecake, syllabub, lemon ice cream and lemon granita (like a sorbet but not whipped, so the ice forms into granules).

MUM'S SWEET TART PASTRY

This pastry is particularly good for fruit tarts, custard tart and treacle tart. One reason why it wins compliments is because lemon acids break down the wheat protein gluten, which helps to make the pastry lovely and light.

275g/10oz/3 cups plain (all-purpose) flour
25g/1oz/¼ cup ground almonds
150g/6oz/1½ sticks cold butter, diced
90g/3oz/heaped ⅓ cup caster (superfine) sugar
1 egg yolk
3 tbsp single (light) cream
zest of ½ lemon

Mix the flour and ground almonds in a large bowl, then quickly rub in (cut in) the butter. Stir in the sugar. In a small bowl, mix the egg yolk with the cream and the lemon zest, then stir this into the mixture and bring it together into a ball. Cover with clingfilm (plastic wrap) and refrigerate for half an hour before rolling out.

LEMON SORBET

Some people like lemon sorbet between courses to 'cleanse the palate' and others prefer it as a dessert. Whatever your choice, the sweet-sharp tang of this frozen concoction is always a refreshing surprise. The limoncello (lemon vodka) adds a slight kick.

225g/8oz/1 cup caster (superfine) sugar
5 or 6 lemons, to give 300ml/10fl oz/1¼ cups juice
2 egg whites
2 tbsp limoncello (optional)

Put the sugar and 570ml/20fl oz/2¼ cups water into a heavy-based pan and stir over a medium heat until the sugar has dissolved. Pare the rind from 3 of the lemons and add it to the pan. Simmer for 10 minutes, then remove the rind and stir in the lemon juice and limoncello, if using. Pour the mixture into a shallow container and freeze for 2 hours, or until mushy.

Remove and stir briskly. Whisk the egg whites until they form stiff peaks and fold into the sorbet. Return to the freezer for 4 hours, or until firm.

Remove from the freezer 30 minutes before serving to allow the sorbet to soften slightly.

LEMON SOUFFLÉ

Aerating cream and lemon juice with beaten egg whites and setting the mixture with gelatine creates a show-stopping dessert. It's particularly dramatic if you set the mixture in a dish with a paper collar. Later, when you remove the collar, the soufflé will tower over the top of the dish.

    4 eggs, separated
    250g/9oz/heaped 1 cup caster (superfine) sugar
    juice and grated zest of 3 lemons
    300ml/10fl oz/1¼ cups double (heavy) cream
    1 sachet (12.5g/½oz) powdered gelatine (unflavoured powdered
      gelatin)

To make a paper collar for a soufflé dish, measure around a tall, straight-sided soufflé dish. Cut a piece of greaseproof paper or baking parchment 10cm/4in longer than the length and 20cm/8in tall. Fold it along its length, then, using paper clips and sticky tape, fix it around the dish so that it stands proud of the top by 8cm/3in. Secure tightly with string.

Put the egg yolks, sugar, lemon zest and lemon juice into a bowl, straining the juice to remove any pulp. Put the bowl over a pan of simmering water and whisk the contents until thick. Remove from the heat and whisk for a further 5 minutes.

In a separate bowl, whip the cream until it begins to thicken and has the consistency of tomato ketchup (catsup), then fold it into the lemon mixture.

Put 150ml/5fl oz/scant ⅔ cup water into a small bowl and sprinkle the gelatine on top. Stand the bowl in a pan containing a little simmering water until the gelatine has completely dissolved and the mixture is clear and light brown. Stir the liquid into the lemon mixture.

Finally, in another bowl, whisk the egg whites until they form stiff peaks, then fold them into the lemon mixture.

Spoon the lemon mixture into the prepared dish and put in the refrigerator to set.

Carefully peel off the paper collar before serving.

LEMON MERINGUE PIE

The meringue topping on this pie has a crisp surface and a soft inside. Its sweetness and combination of textures are dramatic partners for the lemony filling. A favourite way to eat it is cold with thick cream.

FOR THE PASTRY
225g/8oz/1¾ cups plain (all-purpose) flour, plus extra for dusting
100g/3½oz/scant ½ cup cold unsalted butter, diced
2 tsp caster (superfine) sugar
1 egg yolk

FOR THE LEMON FILLING
100g/3½oz/scant ½ cup caster (superfine) sugar
3 tbsp cornflour (cornstarch)
juice and grated zest of 4 lemons
6 egg yolks
100g/3½oz/scant ½ cup unsalted butter, melted

FOR THE MERINGUE
6 egg whites, at room temperature
300g/11oz/1⅓ cups caster (superfine) sugar

To make the pastry, sift the flour into a bowl and quickly rub in (cut in) the butter to form a crumbly mixture. Add the sugar, egg yolk and about 2 tablespoons of cold water and mix – first with a knife, then with your fingers – to form a ball of dough that leaves the sides of the bowl clean. Wrap the dough in cling-film (plastic wrap) and put it in the refrigerator for 30 minutes to rest.

Preheat the oven to 190ºC/375ºF/gas 5. Put a 23cm/9in greased, loose-bottomed tart tin on a baking tray.

On a worktop dusted with flour, roll out the chilled dough into a circle slightly larger than the tin. Lift it carefully into the tin and prick the base with a fork. Cover with a circle of grease-proof paper, baking parchment or aluminium foil, and fill the hollow with ceramic baking beans or dried beans. Trim the excess dough from the sides. Bake for 15 minutes, then remove the paper and beans and continue cooking for another 5 minutes or until the pastry is pale gold and dry. Remove the tin and lower the oven heat to 160ºC/325ºF/gas 3.

To make the lemon filling, put the sugar and cornflour into a bowl and stir in enough cold water to make a paste. Put 50ml/2fl oz water and the lemon zest into a saucepan and bring to the boil. Slowly stir this liquid into the cornflour paste and whisk until smooth. Beat in the egg yolks and melted butter. Return the mixture to the pan and heat gently, stirring, until thickened, then stir in the lemon juice. Pour the mixture into the pastry case.

To make the meringue, put the egg whites into a large clean bowl and whisk to form stiff peaks. Add half the sugar and whisk well, then add the other half and whisk again. Spoon the meringue over the lemon filling so as to cover all the filling, and bake for 25 minutes, or until the meringue is crisp on the outside but still soft inside.

LEMON TART

This pale yellow sweet-sharp tart tastes such a treat that little can beat it. You can pretty it up by using a fluted tart tin, or by putting a paper doily on the top of the cooked and cooled tart before sprinkling it with icing (confectioner's) sugar.

FOR THE PASTRY
200g/7oz/1²/₃ cups plain (all-purpose) flour, sifted
1 tbsp icing (confectioner's) sugar
100g/3½oz/scant ½ cup cold butter, diced
1 egg, beaten

FOR THE FILLING
3 eggs
juice and grated zest of 3 lemons
125g/5oz/heaped ½ cup caster (superfine) sugar
150ml/5fl oz/scant ²/₃ cup double (heavy) cream
juice of 1 orange
4 tbsp sifted icing (confectioner's) sugar, or caster (superfine) sugar

To make the pastry, sift the flour and icing (confectioner's) sugar into a bowl, add the butter and rub it (cut it) in quickly and lightly to form a crumbly mixture. With your hands, mix in enough of the beaten egg to make the mixture stick together in a ball. Wrap the dough in clingfilm (plastic wrap) and put it in the refrigerator for 30 minutes to rest.

Preheat the oven to 180°C/350°F/gas 4. Put a 23cm/9in buttered, loose-bottomed tart tin on a baking tray.

On a worktop dusted with flour, roll the chilled dough out into a circle slightly larger than the tin. Lift it carefully into the tin and prick the base with a fork. Cover with a circle of greaseproof paper, baking parchment or aluminium foil, and fill the hollow with ceramic baking beans or dried beans. Trim the excess dough from the sides. Bake for 20 minutes, then remove the paper and beans and continue cooking for another 10 minutes or until the pastry is pale gold and dry. Remove the tin and lower the oven heat to 160°C/325°F/gas 3.

To make the filling, put the eggs, lemon zest and sugar into a bowl and whisk for 2 minutes. Mix in the cream and the lemon and orange juice, then pour the mixture into the pastry case. Bake for 30–35 minutes or until the filling is just set. Remove from the oven and leave to cool for 5 minutes, then transfer to a plate. When completely cool, dust with the icing (confectioner's) sugar and then caramelize the top either by putting the tart under a hot grill (broiler) or using a cook's blowtorch.

LEMON DELICIOUS

This favourite dessert has various other names – including lemon surprise pudding – reflecting its enduring popularity. As it cooks, the lemony mixture separates into a fluffy sponge set over a light citrus sauce.

> 175g/6oz/¾ cup caster (superfine) sugar
> 75g/3oz/6 tbsp butter, at room temperature
> 4 eggs
> grated zest and juice of 3 lemons
> 50g/2oz/½ cup plain (all-purpose) flour
> 300ml/10fl oz/1¼ cups milk
> sifted icing (confectioner's) sugar, to dust

Preheat the oven to 180ºC/350ºF/gas 4.

Beat the sugar and butter in a bowl until light and fluffy. Beat in the egg yolks one at a time, then stir in the lemon zest and flour. Add the lemon juice and milk, and whisk until smooth.

In a separate bowl, whisk the egg whites until they form soft peaks, then fold them lightly into the lemon mixture. Spoon the mixture into a buttered soufflé dish. Place the dish in a baking tin and pour hot water into the tin so it comes halfway up the sides of the dish.

Bake for 45 minutes, or until the top is light brown and just set when tested with a fine skewer. Dust with sifted icing (confectioner's) sugar.

Bread and Cakes

When incorporating lemon juice and zest into bread and cakes, you can stimulate the tastebuds further by adding other flavours that go well with them, such as herbs (as in herb and lemon bread), almonds (as in lemon almond cakes), polenta (as in lemon polenta cakes), ginger (as in lemon-iced ginger cake) and poppyseeds (as in lemon and poppyseed muffins).

HERB AND LEMON BREAD

We've all heard of garlic bread, but its close cousin – herb and lemon bread – can sometimes be even better. It's particularly good, for example, with grilled (broiled) sardines, smoked salmon or omelettes.

    1 baguette
    100g/3½oz/scant ½ cup butter, softened
    2 tbsp olive oil
    handful of fresh parsley, oregano, basil or other herbs, finely
        chopped
    grated zest of 2 lemons
    pinch of black pepper

Preheat the oven to 200ºC/400ºF/gas 6.
    Cut the bread into slices, but not quite all the way through.
    Put all the remaining ingredients into a bowl and mix well, then spread both sides of each slice of bread with the herb butter. Wrap the bread in aluminium foil, put on a baking tray and heat for 15 to 20 minutes.

LEMON AND POPPYSEED MUFFINS

Combining the flavours of lemon and poppyseeds gives a surprisingly attractive twist to a batch of comforting home-made muffins.

350g/12oz/3½ cups plain (all-purpose) flour
1 tbsp baking powder
125g/5oz/scant ⅔ cup caster (superfine) sugar
2 eggs
180ml/6fl oz/¾ cup milk
1 tsp vanilla extract
4 tbsp corn or other vegetable oil
50g/2oz/4 tbsp butter, melted
grated zest of 1 lemon
2 tbsp poppyseeds

Line a 12-cup muffin tin with paper cases, unless it is nonstick.
Preheat the oven to 180°C/350°F/gas 4.
Sift the flour and baking powder into a bowl and stir in the sugar. Add the eggs, milk, vanilla extract, oil, butter, lemon zest and poppyseeds and beat well. Spoon into the muffin tin and bake for 25 minutes or until golden brown and cooked through.

LEMON POLENTA CAKE

Yellow polenta flour is sometimes sold as 'cornmeal' or 'maize meal' in the UK (where the name 'polenta' is often reserved for the cooked dish of that name, and where cornflour is a fine white powder) and known as 'grits' or 'medium-coarse corn meal' in the USA. It gives these cakes an unusual texture and is good if you want to avoid wheat. The slightly crunchy topping is an optional extra.

250g/9oz/1 cup butter, at room temperature
250g/9oz/heaped 1 cup caster (superfine) sugar, plus
100g/3½oz/scant ½ cup for the topping, if using
175g/6oz/1¾ cups ground almonds
3 eggs
juice and grated zest of 2 lemons
175g/6oz/1¼ cups polenta
1 tsp baking powder

Preheat the oven to 160ºC/325ºF/gas 3. Line a 26 × 16.5cm/10¼ × 6½in baking tin with baking parchment or buttered grease-proof paper.

Put the butter and sugar into a large bowl and beat until light and fluffy. Stir in the ground almonds, then beat in the eggs one by one. Make the juice of the lemons up to 150ml/5fl oz/scant ⅔ cup with water, then fold in with the lemon zest, polenta and baking powder.

Spoon the mixture into the tin and bake for 45–60 minutes until lightly golden and just firm in the centre, so it springs back when pressed gently. Cool completely in the tin, then, if using the topping, sprinkle with the sugar and grill (broil) until the sugar melts and goes light brown. Alternatively, use a cook's blowtorch. Leave the cake in the tin for 1 hour (or the topping will be overly crunchy), then remove and cut into pieces.

LEMON-ICED GINGER CAKE

Lemon and ginger go very well together, and combining these flavours in a cake gives an excellent result.

175g/6oz/¾ cup butter, plus extra for greasing
225g/8oz/1 cup light corn syrup
juice and grated zest of 1 lemon
3 tbsp crystallized ginger, chopped
2 eggs
180ml/6fl oz/¾ cup milk
200g/7oz/1²/₃ cups self-raising flour
½ tsp bicarbonate of soda (baking soda)
1 tsp baking powder
2 tsp ground ginger
pinch of black pepper
100g/3½oz/heaped ¾ cup icing (confectioner's) sugar, sifted

Butter and line with greaseproof paper or baking parchment an 18cm/7in cake tin, or use a nonstick one.

Preheat the oven to 180ºC/350ºF/gas 4.

Put the butter, syrup, lemon zest and crystallized ginger into a saucepan and heat gently until the butter has melted.

Put the eggs and milk into a bowl and whisk. Sift the flour, bicarbonate of soda, baking powder, ground ginger and pepper into a large bowl. Add the egg and milk mixture and beat to a smooth batter.

Pour into the cake tin and bake in the centre of the oven for about 35–40 minutes, or until a skewer pressed into the cake comes out clean. Leave the cake to cool in the tin for 10 minutes, then turn it out onto a wire rack to cool completely.

For the icing, put the icing (confectioner's) sugar into a

bowl, stir in 1 tablespoon of the lemon juice and spread the icing over the cake with a palette knife.

LEMON ALMOND CAKES (FRIANDS)

These gorgeous little cakes have hints of citrus and almond flavours and are perfect with a cup of mid-morning coffee or afternoon tea, or as a dessert along with a spoonful of thick cream. Use a friand tin if you have one.

100g/3½oz/scant ½ cup unsalted butter, plus extra for greasing
3 tbsp plain (all-purpose) flour
100g/3½oz/scant 1 cup icing (confectioner's) sugar, plus more
    for dusting
75g/3oz/⅓ cup ground almonds
3 egg whites
grated zest of 1 lemon
few drops almond essence

Heat the oven to 200°C/400°F/gas 6. Generously butter a 6-cup muffin tin.

Melt the butter and leave to cool.

Sift the flour and icing sugar into a bowl. Add the ground almonds and mix with your fingers.

In another bowl, whisk the egg whites until they become foamy, then stir into the flour and sugar with the lemon zest, almond essence and melted butter.

Spoon the mixture into the muffin tins and bake for 15 minutes or until golden-brown and just firm to the touch. Cool for 5 minutes, then turn out on to a wire rack. Dust lightly with icing sugar.

Other

The enormous variety of recipes that include lemons emphasizes how useful it is to have lemons available in our kitchen. Most of us are familiar with lemonade, lemon curd and lemon marmalade. We may enjoy lemon and parsley stuffing, candied peel and hollandaise sauce. And we're used to sometimes using lemon juice instead of vinegar in a salad dressing. We can also knock up a soothing drink of hot lemon and honey, and may enjoy lemon-flavoured alcoholic drinks, such as a Margarita, whiskey sour or limoncello. But the Italian habit of dressing meat and fish with gremolata, or the Moroccan way of incorporating preserved lemons into casseroles, are less well known. And you may also want to experiment with making your own lemon chutney.

GREMOLATA

Traditionally used in Italy to garnish the veal dish osso bucco, this delightful combination of Mediterranean flavours can also lend a distinctive flourish to other meats, and fish. Make it no longer than 1 hour before it's needed.

  grated zest of 1 lemon
  4 garlic cloves, crushed
  2 handfuls of fresh parsley, chopped

Mix the lemon zest, garlic and parsley in a bowl. Sprinkle over cooked meat, fish or casseroles before serving.

LEMON AND MUSTARD DRESSING

You can vary this dressing by altering the amounts of mustard and honey, by using different oils, by adding herbs (such as chopped marjoram), or – if you like a creamier dressing – by stirring in a little mayonnaise or cream.

  juice and grated zest of 1 lemon
  6 tbsp walnut or olive oil
  1 tsp mustard
  1 tsp clear honey
  pinch of salt
  large pinch of black pepper

Put all the ingredients into a small bowl and mix well; alternatively, put them into a jar with a screw-top lid and shake well.

LEMON 'BLENDER' MAYONNAISE

Using a blender lets you whizz up this lovely lemony mayo very quickly and without the worry that it will curdle. Of course, you could also prepare it with a hand whisk if you prefer.

1 egg
1 tsp mustard
pinch of black pepper
½ tsp sugar
300ml/10fl oz/1¼ cups olive oil
juice of 1 lemon
2 tsp wine vinegar

Put the egg, mustard, pepper, sugar and 4 tablespoons of the olive oil into a blender. Cover and whizz until smooth. Uncover and, with the blender running at medium speed, slowly add 150ml/5fl oz/scant ⅔ cup of the oil plus the lemon juice. Whizz until the mixture is smooth, then slowly add the remaining oil, plus the vinegar. Whizz again until the mayonnaise is thick, then add 4 teaspoons of boiling water and whizz slowly until incorporated.

LEMON AND MUSTARD-SEED CHUTNEY

Opening a jar of homemade chutney is always a treat, and this one goes particularly well with cold ham or lamb and with curries of all sorts.

3 lemons, chopped and pips removed

2 tsp salt

3 small onions, diced

300ml/10fl oz/1¼ cups balsamic vinegar

1 tsp ground mixed spice (apple pie spice)

2 tbsp mustard seeds

225g/8oz/1 cup firmly packed dark muscovado sugar

50g/2oz/½ cup raisins

Put the chopped lemons into a large pan and sprinkle with the salt. Cover with a cloth or kitchen paper and leave for about 10 hours.

Stir in the onions, balsamic vinegar, ground spice, mustard seeds, sugar and raisins. Bring to the boil, then simmer for about 50 minutes or until the chopped lemon is soft.

Meanwhile, sterilize two well-washed 450g/1lb preserving jars or one 900g/2lb jar by boiling the rubber seals in hot water for 10 minutes, and putting the jars themselves into a hot oven for 10 minutes.

Remove the chutney from the heat and ladle into the warmed jars. Put a disc of waxed paper on top of the chutney in each jar, then seal and store in a cool dark place. This chutney can be eaten straight away, but will last for 1 year unopened. Once opened, it will last for up to 2 months if kept in a refrigerator.

PRESERVED LEMONS

The distinctive flavour of preserved lemons is essential for a North African tagine (stew). Salting the lemons softens them and drains away any bitterness, while storing them in oil gives them a delightfully mellow flavour.

15 small unwaxed lemons, washed and sliced
3 tbsp sea salt
2 tsp paprika
4 bay leaves
720ml/24fl oz/3 cups walnut or hazelnut oil

Layer the lemon slices in a colander, sprinkling each layer with salt. Leave for 24 hours, then pat dry with kitchen paper.

Sterilize a 1kg/2lb 4oz well-washed preserving jar by boiling the rubber seal in hot water for 10 minutes, and putting the jar itself into a hot oven for 10 minutes.

Lay the slices in the clean jar, sprinkling each layer with a little paprika and inserting a bay leaf every few layers. Cover generously with oil, cover with a disc of waxed paper, then seal and store in a cool dark place. The lemons can be eaten straight away, but will last for 2 years unopened. Once opened, they will keep for 6 months in a refrigerator.

LEMON CURD

This delightful lemony concoction is a favourite when spread on scones, bread, waffles or pancakes.

125g/5oz/½ cup unsalted butter
220g/7oz/1 cup caster (superfine) sugar
juice and grated zest of 2–3 lemons (to give 120ml/4fl oz/½ cup
   juice)
6 egg yolks

Sterilize a well-washed 450g/1lb preserving jar by boiling its rubber seal in hot water for 10 minutes, and putting the jar itself into a hot oven for 10 minutes.

Melt the butter in a heavy-based saucepan and whisk in the sugar and lemon juice and zest. Add the egg yolks and whisk until smooth. Heat gently, stirring, for 10–15 minutes or until thick enough to coat the back of a wooden spoon. Cook for a further 2 minutes, without boiling, then remove from the heat.

Pour the curd into the warmed jar, cover with a disc of waxed paper and seal tightly. Leave to cool at room temperature, then refrigerate. Alternatively, keep the curd in a covered container in the refrigerator for up to 3 weeks or in the freezer for up to 2 months.

LEMONADE 1

Home-made lemonade is always a winner. It's also easy to make, and if you have a blender you can prepare it in hardly any time at all. Drink warm in winter or to soothe a cold, and cold in summer.

> 3 lemons, sliced and pips removed
> 100g/3½oz/scant ½ cup caster (superfine) sugar
> a few ice cubes (optional)

With a blender: Put the lemon slices, sugar and 570ml/20fl oz/2¼ cups just-boiled water into a blender and whizz until smooth. Stir in the same amount of water again. Strain the lemonade into a jug. Drink the lemonade while still warm, or let it cool, then add a few ice cubes before serving.

Without a blender: Put the lemon slices and sugar into a jug. Add 1.1l/40fl oz/4½ cups just-boiled water and stir until the sugar has dissolved, pressing the lemons against the side of the jug to extract the maximum flavour. Strain the lemonade into a jug. Drink the lemonade while still warm, or let it cool and add a few ice cubes before serving.

LEMONADE 2

This recipe leaves out the lemon pith, making it less bitter than the recipe above.

> zest (grated or in strips) and juice of 3 lemons
> 100g/3½oz/scant ½ cup caster (superfine) sugar
> ice cubes

Put the lemon zest and juice into a jug, add the sugar and 1.1 l/2 pints/4½ cups just-boiled water and stir until the sugar has dissolved. Strain the lemonade into a jug. Drink the lemonade while still warm, or let it cool and add the ice cubes before serving.

LEMON BARLEY WATER

This variation of lemonade is not only delicious but is also said to promote health.

  75g/3oz/⅓ cup pot (unpearled) barley (barley with its husk and
    bran removed), washed
  3 lemons, chopped
  50g/2oz/¼ cup light brown sugar

Put the barley and 1.7 l/3 pints/7 cups just-boiled water in a pan. Bring to the boil, then cover and simmer for 30 minutes. Add the chopped lemons and sugar and leave to cool. Strain the lemonade into a jug and serve. This drink can be kept in a refrigerator for up to 5 days.

LEMON TEA

Simply add a couple of lemon slices or a few wide slivers of lemon zest to a cup or mug of hot black Indian tea, then sweeten the tea with sugar if desired.

HOT PUNCH

The bitter tannins from the tea and red wine complement the sweetness of the orange, honey and sugar, while the citrus notes of the lemon and the spiciness of the cinnamon and cloves add to the fragrant bouquet of this party drink.

2 teabags
juice and pared zest of 1 lemon
juice and pared zest of 1 orange
1 cinnamon stick
2 cloves
570ml/20fl oz/2¼ cups cups red wine
2 tbsp clear honey
1 tbsp sugar

Put the teabags into a large bowl or jug, add 1.2l/2 pints/5 cups just-boiled water and leave to infuse for 20 minutes. Add the lemon and orange zest to the tea, then add both juices plus the cinnamon stick and cloves, and stir. Strain the liquid through a fine sieve into a large pan. Add the wine, honey and sugar and heat, stirring.

WHISKEY SOUR AND OTHER 'SOURS'

Alcoholic drinks containing lemon or other citrus juice are sometimes called 'sours'. You can vary the following recipe by using another spirit (such as gin, white rum, vodka or tequila) instead of the whiskey, or by using a liqueur (such as Cointreau or amaretto) instead of the whiskey and sugar syrup. Note that 1 cocktail measure is 25ml/1¼fl oz or 1½ tablespoons.

  1 measure lemon juice
  ½ measure sugar syrup
  2 measures whiskey
  crushed ice
  Maraschino cherry, half a lemon slice or 1–3 strips of lemon zest
  (optional), to decorate

Shake the lemon juice, sugar syrup, whiskey and crushed ice in a cocktail shaker, then pour into a glass. Decorate, if desired, with a cherry, half lemon slice or zest.

Useful Websites

Here are some of the organizations concerned with lemons and lemon products around the world.

United Kingdom

Global Orange Groves UK
globalorangegroves.co.uk
This nursery offers a variety of citrus trees, including several types of lemon, that are suitable for growing in the UK.

United States

USDA (United States Department of Agriculture)
www.usda.gov
Provides information on lemons and lemon juice.

Florida Citrus Information
www.UltimateCitrus.com
Provides links to various sites associated with the citrus industry in Florida.

Australia

Citrus Australia (formerly Australian Citrus Growers)
www.citrusaustralia.com.au
Represents citrus growers in Australia.

New Zealand

New Zealand Citrus Growers Incorporated
www.citrus.co.nz
Promotes the interests of citrus growers and the sustainable
growth and profitability of the citrus industry in New
Zealand.

Argentina

Tucuman Citrus Association
www.atcitrus.com/english
Represents the citrus industry in Argentina, including
producers, packers, manufacturers and exporters.

South Africa

Citrus Growers Association of Southern Africa
www.cga.co.za
Represents producers of export citrus fruit throughout
Southern Africa, including Zimbabwe and Swaziland.

Index